WALKING BROOKLYN

30 Tours Exploring Historical Legacies, Neighborhood Culture, Side Streets, and Waterways

Second Edition

Adrienne Onofri

WILDERNESS PRESS . . . *on the trail since 1967*

Walking Brooklyn: 30 Tours Exploring Historical Legacies, Neighborhood Culture, Side Streets, and Waterways

Second edition, first printing

Copyright © 2017 by Adrienne Onofri

Project editor: Ritchey Halphen
Cartography and cover design: Scott McGrew
Interior design: Annie Long
Photos: Adrienne Onofri
Copy editor: Erin Mahoney Harris
Proofreader: Rebecca Henderson
Indexer: Sylvia Coates

Library of Congress Cataloging-in-Publication Data

Names: Onofri, Adrienne, author.
Title: Walking Brooklyn : 30 tours exploring historical legacies, neighborhood culture, side streets, and
    waterways / Adrienne Onofri.
Description: Second edition. | Birmingham, AL : Wilderness Press, 2017. | Includes index.
Identifiers: LCCN 2017015019| ISBN 978-0-89997-803-1 (pbk.) | ISBN 978-0-89997-804-8 (e-book)
Subjects: LCSH: Brooklyn (New York, N.Y.)—Tours. | Walking—New York (State)—New York—
    Guidebooks. | Brooklyn (New York, N.Y.)—Guidebooks | New York (N.Y.)—Guidebooks.
Classification: LCC F129.B7 O56 2017 | DDC 917.47/2304—dc23
LC record available at lccn.loc.gov/2017015019

Published by 🐾 **WILDERNESS PRESS**
An imprint of AdventureKEEN
2204 First Ave. S., Suite 102
Birmingham, AL 35233
800-443-7227, fax 205-326-1012

Visit wildernesspress.com for a complete list of our books and for ordering information. Contact us at our website, at facebook.com/wildernesspress1967, or at twitter.com/wilderness1967 with questions or comments. To find out more about who we are and what we're doing, visit blog.wildernesspress.com.

Distributed by Publishers Group West

Cover photo: Brooklyn Bridge Park and the Manhattan Bridge (Walk 1, page 2)

Frontispiece: Elegant rowhouses on Stuyvesant Avenue in Bedford-Stuyvesant (Walk 20, page 122)

Page 134: sculpture by Sung Ha No; *page 162:* mural by Nicer Tats Cru. Both appear in this book with the permission of the artists.

SAFETY NOTICE Although Wilderness Press and Adrienne Onofri have made every attempt to ensure that the information in this book is accurate at press time, they are not responsible for any loss, damage, injury, or inconvenience that may occur to anyone while using this book. You are responsible for your own safety and health while following the walking trips described here.

Acknowledgments

If I were to name names, I might inadvertently leave someone out. So, to everybody who provided me with assistance or answers, a great big *thanks*—for that contribution and for your contribution to the life and culture of Brooklyn. Thank you to the Wilderness Press/AdventureKEEN team for their support and patience. This book is dedicated in memory of my mother, who passed away while it was in production—a proud New Yorker, she instilled my curiosity and affection for the city. Finally, thanks and kisses to Daniel, my husband and favorite fact-checker.

Author's Note

Try as I might, I cannot include *every* place that's interesting, eye-catching, or otherwise worthy of note in a book that must be light enough to carry around as you walk. I encourage you to make your own discoveries to supplement what I share on these tours. Look at buildings I don't describe, examine ornamentation on buildings, read historic markers and interpretive signs I haven't pointed out, check out eateries and shops . . . you're bound to see things that I had to omit to keep the book portable. While I do mention some restaurants and bars, I leave it to you to find what appeals to your taste (I also avoided extensive restaurant and bar coverage in the interest of keeping the book current). Consult blogs, message boards, and guidebooks for recommendations.

Also seek out information online about special events like music festivals, historic-house tours, artists' open-studio weekends, and free outdoor performances and screenings, as well as the weekly and seasonal food, vintage, and/or artisan markets (Brooklyn Flea and Smorgasburg chief among them). They're a great way to enhance your experience in a neighborhood. If you plan to visit museums, historic sites, or galleries, check in advance when they're open—some have limited hours, and even the major ones aren't open seven days a week.

On most of these routes, you pass subway and bus stops, so you can curtail a tour and do the rest of it another time. Pick up a Brooklyn bus map (available free at most subway stations), see it online at mta.info/nyct/maps/busbkln.pdf, or use an NYC transit app for guidance in such situations. A neighborhood map—on paper or your phone—will come in handy in case you wish to veer off-course to see something that catches your fancy. You're in the most walkable of cities, so get yourself some comfortable shoes and have fun!   —*Adrienne Onofri*

Table of Contents

Walking Brooklyn

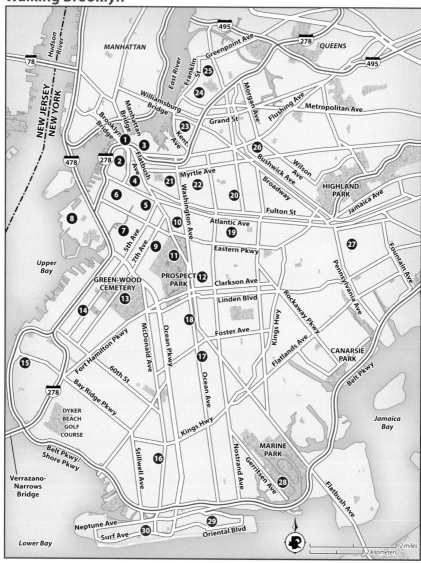

Numbers on this overview map correspond to walk numbers. A map for each tour follows the text for that walk.

Introduction

When *Walking Brooklyn* was first published in 2007, Brooklyn was on the brink of change. Yet nobody could have foreseen just how far-reaching and momentous that change would be. It's a renaissance unprecedented in modern urban history, and it entails so much more than skyscraper construction, waterfront development, or gentrification spreading from one neighborhood to the next. Brooklyn has emerged as a worldwide locus of trendy, artisanal cool and a wellspring of artistic, culinary, and technological creativity. It has become, in the words of *New York* magazine, New York City's "most dominant cultural export." Brooklyn went into this a place and came out a brand name. And, occasionally, a punchline, as that amalgam of qualities now synonymous with the word *Brooklyn*—hip, highly educated, cross-cultural, environmentally responsible, haute rustic, retro-influenced—is parodied nearly as much as it's imitated.

Yet while this renaissance has renewed hometown pride, it also has perpetuated a disconnect between today's Brooklyn and the Brooklyn of so many cherished 20th-century memories, and between the "new" Brooklyn and the sizable swath of this 40-neighborhood, 2.6 million–person borough that hasn't really changed. A lot of newer Brooklynites grew up far from Kings County. They may not even know they're supposed to hate Walter O'Malley for banishing the Dodgers to California, or Robert Moses for bulldozing a highway through their streets. Earlier events—from the devastating assault by the King's army during the Revolutionary War, to the high-bourgeois Victorian age, to the lurid decline of the 1970s—have left their mark on Brooklyn. So we have a place defined by both the past and the future, a personality both nostalgic and on the cutting edge.

Brooklyn has the unique history of having been an independent city, and before that was composed of several different cities and townships. It can also boast of the great outdoors, with parks and community gardens galore and a shoreline that stretches from river to bay to ocean. These walks aim to capture all this diversity in Brooklyn's geography, history, and people. I hope you have fun exploring and are enlightened and excited along the way.

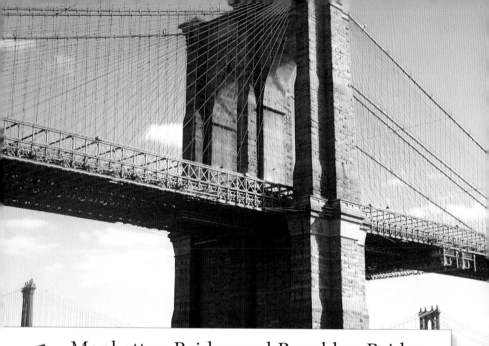

1 Manhattan Bridge and Brooklyn Bridge:
In One, Out the Other

Above: One of America's proudest architectural achievements, the Brooklyn Bridge

BOUNDARIES: Canal St. (Manhattan), Jay St., Cadman Plaza Park, ferry landing
DISTANCE: 4.1 miles
SUBWAY: B or D at Grand St. (Manhattan)

Standing less than half a mile apart, the Brooklyn and Manhattan Bridges span the East River between two downtowns: lower Manhattan and the neighborhood known as Downtown Brooklyn. Both bridges had long, complicated, controversial journeys to completion, and both set precedents in design and construction. The Manhattan, opened in 1909, ushered in an age of lighter and narrower suspension bridges, whose deck and cables could deflect weight and wind forces enough to decrease reliance on clunky-looking girders. But the Brooklyn Bridge, dating to 1883, was an engineering marvel, and now it's also revered as a work of art. While the Manhattan Bridge has neither the iconic status nor aesthetic cachet of the Brooklyn Bridge, together they create a striking image and apt symbol of this city that's always on the move.

Walk Description

Begin in Manhattan at Canal Street and the Bowery. Go onto the plaza for an up-close view of the Manhattan Bridge's grandiose entrance. The crosswalk from the south side of the plaza leads right onto the bridge's pedestrian lane. Because Manhattan Bridge pedestrians have just one "caged" lane, as opposed to an entire level on the Brooklyn Bridge, this is a more confining walk. But it offers its own unique experiences—like walking beside the subway train (which clamors across the bridge mere feet away) and possibly even feeling the bridge's vibrations.

After walking down the steps from the bridge on the Brooklyn side, go to the right. You're on Jay Street and entering Dumbo, a neighborhood given new life by artists and entrepreneurs a century after its industrial heyday and one of NYC's priciest. It's even spawned a Dumbo Heights—the group of buildings in this vicinity connected by sky bridges. Now office, retail, and hotel space, the buildings until recently had belonged to the Jehovah's Witnesses, who've moved upstate after a century headquartered in this part of Brooklyn.

Cross Jay Street at Sands Street, then turn around (with the bridge to your left): that gold-domed building you see three blocks up Jay is St. James, not a church but a "minor papal basilica," per the Vatican. It is the mother church of Brooklyn for Catholics; before St. James was established in 1822, Catholics who lived anywhere on Long Island had to travel to Manhattan for services (the current building dates to 1903). Now turn back, cross Sands, and go to the left.

Turn right on Pearl Street. Pay a quick visit to the global headquarters of ❶ Etsy to your left on Prospect Street. There are public galleries in the lobby where products designed by Etsy members are displayed. Back on Pearl, continue downhill. Traffic might be noisy, but it's definitely a cool experience walking through one of the stone arches that support a bridge carrying upward of 80,000 vehicles a day. Plus, you've got cobblestone for ambience once you're past York Street!

Past Front Street, walk across the painted-ground plaza and onto Anchorage Place. Go into the Archway on your left—depending on the day and season, you'll find food vendors, the Brooklyn Flea market, or an event such as a live performance or yoga class.

Resume walking on Anchorage Place. At Plymouth Street, cross over onto Adams Street and walk one block to John Street, where you enter ❷ Brooklyn Bridge Park on your left. You can learn about the area's history and ecology from signs throughout the park. Proceed on the path closest to the water. Be sure to turn around for a great view of the Williamsburg Bridge. After passing under the Manhattan Bridge, you'll reach a couple of picture-perfect spots for gazing at the Brooklyn Bridge and Manhattan skyline, including a pebbly cove with bleacher seating.

After passing the cove, follow the path to the right, leading you to Plymouth Street and Main Street—beneath the Clocktower Building you've seen along the route. Across from it is an immense

Civil War–era warehouse called the Empire Stores, recently rehabbed for offices and retail. Originally built for the world's first commercial coffee-roasting facility, the Empire Stores now features a public atrium and roof deck, eateries, and a Brooklyn Historical Society museum.

Walk between the Empire Stores and the river to ❸ Jane's Carousel, a restored 1922 charmer. Then head to the smaller brick building next to the Empire Stores, ❹ St. Ann's Warehouse, an acclaimed avant-garde theater. Prior to its renovation for St. Ann's, the 1860s-era former tobacco warehouse had been entirely roofless. Walk through the still-roofless public courtyard and come out at the other end on New Dock Street.

Go right on Water Street and follow it to the Fulton Ferry Landing. Two events that shaped the future of the city and the country occurred here. In 1776 George Washington massed 9,500 troops for a furtive evacuation in rowboats and schooners across a river filled with British warships. The Americans had just been routed in the Battle of Long Island, aka the Battle of Brooklyn, and the retreat prevented a complete defeat by the British—and thus saved the fledgling nation. Then, in 1814, Robert Fulton launched his steamboat from here, opening up travel between Brooklyn and Manhattan.

Casual dining abounds at the ferry landing, including in a former fireboat house and old smokestack building (plus, the Michelin-starred River Café is situated beneath the bridge). While you're gaping at the Manhattan skyline, look down at the metal railing around the pier to read a passage from Walt Whitman's poem "Crossing Brooklyn Ferry." Also note ❺ Bargemusic, which features classical concerts year-round inside a barge permanently moored at the ferry landing. This intimate setting offers sharp acoustics unlike those of cavernous auditoriums, and you can see lower Manhattan twinkling from your seat and feel the vessel rocking softly as you listen to world-class artists play.

Head up Old Fulton Street. The buildings to your left were constructed between 1835 and 1839 when the ferry service gave rise to a commercial center (the corner Shake Shack building was originally a hotel). The Eagle Warehouse & Storage Company's fortress on your right was built in 1892, replacing the offices of the *Brooklyn Eagle,* a newspaper that had employed a crusading journalist named Walt Whitman from 1846 to 1848. Back on your left, the white palazzo with a diagonally sited doorway at 1 Front Street was constructed for a bank in 1869. It's made of cast iron, probably for fireproofing. There may be a line outside Grimaldi's, which for years was lauded as the city's best pizza. But the man responsible for its reputation has sold the restaurant and opened Juliana's next door.

Stay to the right to continue up Old Fulton Street, but take note of 5–7 Front Street next to Grimaldi's. It dates to 1834 and is considered the city's oldest surviving office building. Cross Hicks and then Henry Street before Old Fulton becomes Cadman Plaza West.

At Middagh Street, enter ❻ **Cadman Plaza Park** on your left. Walk around to the front of the monument: a bust of William Jay Gaynor, backed by bronze bas-reliefs representing law, strength, and knowledge. During Gaynor's 1910–13 term as mayor of New York, the Brooklynite walked from his Park Slope home to City Hall via the Brooklyn Bridge.

With your back to Gaynor, follow the path and then go up the steps to the front of the World War II memorial—an enormous limestone rectangle flanked by 24-foot-tall statues facing a tree-lined mall. The man represents the battlefield; the woman, home and hearth. Follow the sidewalk or path along the east (woman's) side of the park to the bridge access steps on your left just before Prospect Street.

Once upon a time not too long ago, walking the Brooklyn Bridge was an insider tip you'd give tourists. Not anymore. It can get packed with sightseers, and there are a lot more bicyclists too. Stay in the lane designated for pedestrians. When the Brooklyn Bridge opened in May 1883, it was the tallest structure in the United States and the longest suspension bridge in the world. This wooden-planked promenade was the world's highest human-made observation platform at the time. Today it remains one of the only places in the world where airplanes can fly above people walking above vehicles driving above boats sailing above trains running (through the underwater subway tunnel). Look for a plaque on the Manhattan-facing side of the Brooklyn tower honoring Emily Roebling, who supervised construction of the bridge after her husband, chief engineer Washington Roebling, was paralyzed with the bends (his father John had designed the bridge but died before construction began). The bends—then simply labeled "decompression sickness"—killed 20 men on the bridge construction crew, and others also suffered respiratory and neurological ailments from working inside caissons, the huge airtight chambers installed in the riverbed so men could work underwater laying the foundations. Those caissons, as well as John Roebling's steel "rope" design, were among the bridge's many significant innovations. It dates to a time when one in four bridges would collapse; almost no other American bridge its age is still functional. You can learn about the construction step-by-step from engraved tablets at the railing in the areas around the two towers; they also cover Brooklyn's maritime heritage, East River bridges and islands, and other relevant topics.

This walk may be the ultimate NYC photo op, but the bridge itself is a beloved subject of photographers, painters, poets, filmmakers, and so on. My favorite quote about this experience comes from historian David McCullough, reflecting in the Ken Burns documentary *Brooklyn Bridge:* "The bridge makes one feel better about being alive. I think it makes you glad that you're part of the human community, that you're part of a specie that could create such a structure."

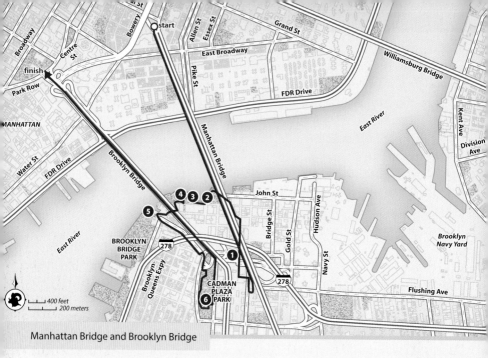

Manhattan Bridge and Brooklyn Bridge

Points of Interest

1. **Etsy** 117 Prospect St.; etsy.com
2. **Brooklyn Bridge Park** Plymouth Street and Adams Street; brooklynbridgepark.org
3. **Jane's Carousel** Brooklyn Bridge Park, Old Dock Street off Water Street; 718-222-2502, janescarousel.com
4. **St. Ann's Warehouse** 45 Water St.; 718-834-8794, stannswarehouse.org
5. **Bargemusic** Fulton Ferry Landing, Water Street and Old Fulton Street; bargemusic.org
6. **Cadman Plaza Park** Cadman Plaza West and Middagh Street; nycgovparks.org

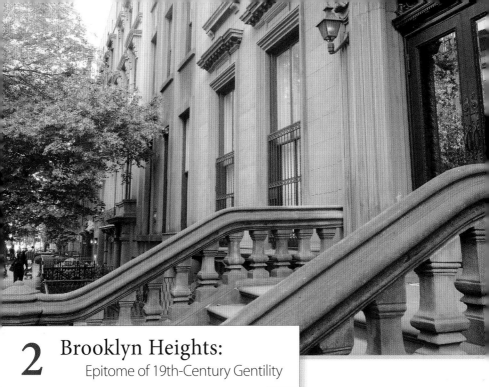

2 Brooklyn Heights:
Epitome of 19th-Century Gentility

Above: *Classic Italianate brownstones on Remsen Street*

BOUNDARIES: Middagh St., Clinton St., State St., Promenade
DISTANCE: 2.5 miles
SUBWAY: 2 or 3 to Clark St.

It may be self-defeating for me to say so, but you really don't need a guide in Brooklyn Heights. It's compact, and wherever you might wander, you'll probably like what you see. This was Brooklyn's first residential neighborhood—America's first suburb, some call it—and it still contains hundreds of antebellum homes. It was also the first historic district designated by the city, which means the old houses haven't been getting demolished, as happens in communities without landmark protection. The architectural riches of Brooklyn Heights include some glorious churches and other public buildings. And perched along its west end is the Promenade, offering views of the East River and many of NYC's most famous landmarks. All things considered, the Heights has few peers among urban communities in this country.

Walk Description

Exit the subway on Henry Street. You've emerged from within the St. George, a hotel described in a 1930s guidebook as "the social mecca of all Brooklyn." It opened in 1885, and by 1929 had expanded to 2,632 guest rooms—the most of any hotel in the world. Its ballroom, saltwater pool, and rooftop restaurant were legendary. The hotel closed in the 1970s, and the building is now residential.

Go to the left on Henry, then make a left on Orange Street. ❶ **Plymouth Church,** on your right, was a destination unto itself from 1849 to 1887, when people came from far and near for the sermons of Congregationalist minister Henry Ward Beecher. Beecher, brother of *Uncle Tom's Cabin* author Harriet Beecher Stowe, was a leading progressive and huge celebrity in his day, complete with his own adultery scandal (the Pulitzer Prize–winning 2006 biography of him is titled *The Most Famous Man in America*). In the garden next to the church are a statue of Beecher (holding one of his mock slave auctions that essentially bought the slave's freedom) and a bas-relief of Abraham Lincoln, who worshipped at the church; both were made by Mount Rushmore sculptor Gutzon Borglum.

Make a right on Hicks Street. That two-dormered corner building on your left at Cranberry dates to 1822.

Turn right on Cranberry Street. Midblock on the left is the Church of the Assumption, erected in 1908. The parish (est. 1842) lost its original building, located farther east, to eminent domain when the Manhattan Bridge was constructed. The Art Deco Cranlyn apartment building on your right near the end of the block has terrific polychromatic terra cotta panels and a metal bas-relief at the main entrance featuring the Williamsburgh Savings Bank clocktower—the pride of Brooklyn at the time of the Cranlyn's construction, as it had opened just a few years earlier as the borough's only skyscraper.

Turn left on Henry. The residential complex to your right, Whitman Close, was the approximate location of the Rome brothers' print shop, where Walt Whitman set type in 1855 for his first edition of *Leaves of Grass.*

Turn left on Middagh Street. On your right is the old factory of Peaks Mason Mints; some of their candies are today produced by the Tootsie Roll company, while their building is now a condo. This block also contains a house from 1829 at #56. Virtually the entire block past Hicks is composed of pre-1850 wood houses. The most celebrated is the corner house at #24, sometimes erroneously identified as the oldest in the Heights (it's close, built in 1824). On the Willow Street side, you can see that the home has its own cottage. Proceed across Willow and look into the playground named for "Cat's in the Cradle" singer Harry Chapin, who grew up in the Heights. Another popular story-song of his, "Taxi," is represented in the benches. Walk around the park, going left onto Columbia Heights.

Make a left on Cranberry. This is the street where Cher kicked a can as she dreamily strolled home after her night at the opera in *Moonstruck*. The house at #19 was used for exterior shots of her home.

Turn right on Willow Street, where the star is #70—built in 1839 and one of the largest Greek Revival homes in New York. Truman Capote wrote *Breakfast at Tiffany's* there while he was the basement tenant of his friend Oliver Smith, a Broadway set designer, who owned the house for 40 years.

On your left after Pineapple the whole block is consumed by an exquisite building that used to be Brooklyn's most expensive hotel, the Leverich Towers, which charged $3 a night in 1931. In the glory days of the Leverich, its towers were illuminated every evening. But in the daylight you can better appreciate their hexagonal design, colonnades, and balconies.

The next block of Willow presents a long and lovely assortment of decorating schemes and eras. One brownstone on your right houses ❷ **Dansk Sømandskirke** (Danish Seamen's Church), the only church in North America that still holds services in Danish. On #110 and 112, look for child figures in the terra cotta decoration, then look all the way up to whoever that is lurking atop #115. Farther down, #155–159 were built in the 1820s, before the current street pattern, which is why they don't align with Willow as the other houses do. Playwright Arthur Miller wrote *The Crucible* while living at #155.

Turn right on Pierrepont Street and then left on Pierrepont Place. The huge Italianate brownstone manses on your right date to 1857: #2 was the childhood home of Alfred Tredway White, who inherited his father's business but ultimately devoted himself to social reform; #3 was built for A. A. Low, an über-successful importer of tea and silk from Asia, whose son Seth grew up to be the only person ever to serve as mayor of both Brooklyn and New York City. Continue across Montague Street onto Montague Terrace, and read of its literary heritage from the plaques on #1 and 5.

Turn right on Remsen Street, walk a short block, and go up the ramp to the ❸ **Brooklyn Heights Promenade.** Stroll as much as you'd like on the Promenade (you'll be exiting at Montague Street); it extends about a third of a mile to Orange Street. With wonderful views and benches all along the way, it is beloved by photographers, canoodlers, and dog walkers alike. For decades the Promenade overlooked abandoned piers and inaccessible waterfront, but now Brooklyn Bridge Park unfolds below you. You can visit it at the end of this walk (see page 12).

Leave the Promenade at Montague, pausing to read the historic marker on a boulder facing the street. At the right corner with Pierrepont Place, the Romanesque #62 was designed by Montrose Morris, architect of several landmark residences (mostly in Bedford-Stuyvesant). Continuing along Montague, watch on your left for a long building with a stepped gable, the Heights Casino. When it was built in 1904, the word *casino* was used for places of various social amusements, not just gambling. This casino was, and is, a renowned racquet club, producing many squash champions and containing the United States' first indoor tennis courts.

On your right after you cross Hicks is the Bossert. From 1909 to 1949, it operated as Hotel Bossert, once lauded as "the Waldorf-Astoria of Brooklyn." Across the street, find the Montague at #105, followed a couple of doors down by the adjoining Berkeley and Grosvenor. All three were designed in 1885 by the Parfitt Brothers, who were responsible for many fine churches and homes in late-19th-century Brooklyn.

From these Queen Anne gems, proceed past Henry and down the block to the 1847 Gothic Revival masterpiece of St. Ann and the Holy Trinity. The church's superb stained-glass windows were the first such windows made in America, and its tower was originally 295 feet—taller than any other structure in Brooklyn or Manhattan—but was eventually shortened to less than half that height because upkeep was so expensive and the rector felt church steeples were being overshadowed by skyscrapers.

Two of the banks that gave Montague Street the nickname "the Wall Street of Brooklyn" stand opposite the church: to your right on Montague is the former Franklin Trust Company (1891), robustly punctuated with dormers and now restored as luxury apartments. Across Clinton Street, Chase occupies a 1915 building that was modeled on a palace in Verona, Italy.

Turn left on Clinton. Next to the church, smile at the faces of Michelangelo, Beethoven, Gutenberg, and Shakespeare—none of whom ever made it to Brooklyn, far as I know—high up on the 1881 building of the ❹ Brooklyn Historical Society (BHS).

Make a left on Pierrepont Street, walking around this Queen Anne landmark with deluxe terra cotta ornamentation. On this side you'll find busts of Benjamin Franklin and Christopher Columbus between window arches. BHS, founded as the Long Island Historical Society, mounts exhibitions and owns an invaluable archive and library of books, maps, correspondence, newspapers, census and landholding records, and other materials. Across from the Historical Society is St. Ann's, a progressive private school. Its building was erected in 1906 as a clubhouse for the well-heeled gentlemen who belonged to the prestigious Crescent Athletic Club.

At the next corner on your right, the Unitarian Church is the oldest church building in Brooklyn. Designed shortly before Holy Trinity by the same architect, Minard Lafever, it helped launch the Gothic Revival movement in the United States with its 1844 construction. The church installed eight Tiffany stained-glass windows for its golden anniversary.

Continue on Pierrepont just past Henry so you can get a good look at the mansion on the left corner. This Romanesque treasure, marred only by a canopy added in the mid–20th century, was completed in 1890 for manufacturing tycoon Herman Behr (whose son Karl, an attorney and tennis

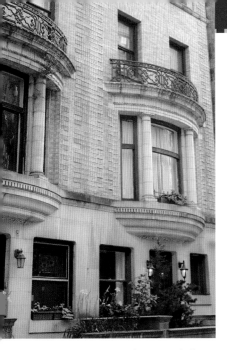
The Pierrepont Street townhouses with these bay windows are steps from the Promenade

champion, would survive the *Titanic*). Check out the dragons fronting the stone porch.

Walk on Henry Street beside the Behr mansion and then cross Montague. You don't need to be close to ❺ **Our Lady of Lebanon Maronite Catholic Cathedral** to spot its Rapunzel tower, but you do want to go up to the entrances on both Henry and Remsen to see its engraved bronze doors—salvage from the *Normandie,* the largest ocean liner in the world, which was being refitted for military deployment during World War II when it caught fire at the dock in Manhattan and capsized. The building was erected in the 1840s for a Congregational church; its Romanesque style was uncharacteristic for its architect, Gothic master Richard Upjohn.

With the church on your right, walk on Remsen. See the "cultural medallion" on #91 about a former resident. Why such a short tenancy here for Henry Miller? He was evicted because he couldn't make rent. The mansion two doors down has a copper roof and may be the standout of this outstanding block.

Turn left on Hicks Street, taking note of Grace Court Alley to your left, a mews of former carriage houses for the mansions on Joralemon and Remsen. On your right at Grace Court, Grace Church proffers another bold design by Richard Upjohn, this one in his more typical Gothic Revival vernacular.

Walk down Grace Court, a tranquil, secluded street with a fantastic view of Manhattan and the Statue of Liberty at the dead end. There's also a celebrity connection: Arthur Miller wrote *Death of a Salesman* at #31, and then sold the house to civil rights leader W. E. B. DuBois.

Return to Hicks and go right.

Make a right on Joralemon. The 1847 brownstone on your left at #58 has blackened windows because there's nothing in the house except a ventilation shaft for the subway.

Turn left on Willow Place. About halfway down the block you find the Unitarian Church's former chapel on your right. Alfred Tredway White, the philanthropic scion who grew up on Pierrepont Place, was its patron. It had to be sold upon his death in 1921 and for a while housed a brothel

Brooklyn Bridge Park

Brooklyn Bridge Park opened in phases starting in 2010 and became one of the city's most popular green spaces in no time. Once you start roaming through the park, you'd never believe this real estate went neglected and inaccessible for so long. Stretching 1.3 miles from Atlantic Avenue (just south of Joralemon) all the way to beneath the Manhattan Bridge, the park centers on five redeveloped piers. At Joralemon Street's Pier 5 are a marina and a picnic area with barbecue grills. Pier 6 features volleyball courts and play-grounds, while the absent Pier 4 has been replaced with a sandy beach and tidal pools. Pier 2 offers shuffle-board, roller skating, and kayaking, while Piers 1 and 3 both have terraces made from salvaged granite. And don't miss the Squibb Park bridge, which carries pedestrians between the park and the foot of Middagh Street. There are lawns, pathways, plantings, and of course views throughout the park, as well as a series of 20- to 30-foot grassy hills that reduce noise level from the nearby expressway. You can also catch a ferry here. Park signage points you where you want to go and shares key historical and environmental information. All facilities and programs are subject to seasonal closings.

frequented by Navy Yard employees. Rescued by a citizens' rehabilitation campaign in the 1960s, it is now used by the Heights Players, a long-running community theater. Toward the end of the block on your left is a group of brick townhouses in a so-called colonnade row. An identical quartet was built directly across the street (both in the 1840s), but it has only one weathered survivor.

Make a right on State Street. The ❻ **park** on your left was renamed for the Beastie Boys' Adam "MCA" Yauch in 2013, one year after his death at age 47. "Born and bred in Brooklyn the U.S.A.," Yauch rapped in "No Sleep Till Brooklyn." He'd learned to ride a bike in this park.

Turn right on Columbia Place, site of one of Alfred T. White's projects, Riverside, partway down on your left. Built in 1890, they were conceived as "model tenements" that elevated the quality of housing that the working class could afford, with decent plumbing and ventilation—not to mention decent aesthetics.

Back at Joralemon, you can go to the left and walk under the highway and across Furman Street to Brooklyn Bridge Park (see sidebar). Or if you'd rather save that for another time, go right on Joralemon and left on Clinton to the R train, about 0.4 mile away.

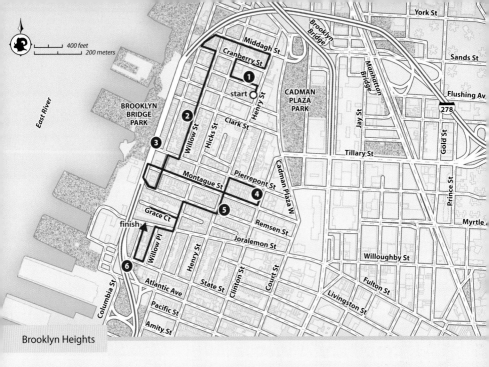

Brooklyn Heights

Points of Interest

1 **Plymouth Church** 57 Orange St.; 718-624-4743, plymouthchurch.org

2 **Dansk Sømandskirke (Danish Seamen's Church)** 102 Willow St.; 718-875-0042, dskny.org

3 **Brooklyn Heights Promenade** West of Columbia Heights between Remsen Street and Orange Street

4 **Brooklyn Historical Society** 128 Pierrepont St., 718-222-4111; brooklynhistory.org

5 **Our Lady of Lebanon Maronite Catholic Cathedral** 113 Remsen St.; 718-624-7228, ololc.org

6 **Adam Yauch Park** State Street and Columbia Place; nycgovparks.org

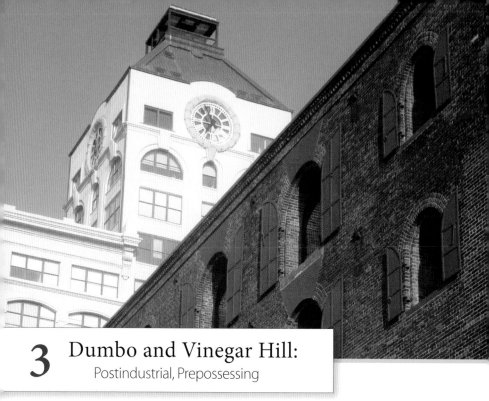

3 Dumbo and Vinegar Hill:
Postindustrial, Prepossessing

BOUNDARIES: Brooklyn Bridge Park, Navy Yard, Sands St., Main St.
DISTANCE: 2 miles
SUBWAY: F to York St.

At a community meeting sometime in the late 1970s, the folks who'd started to repopulate a neglected industrial district on the East River came up with a name for their neighborhood: Dumbo, an acronym for "down under the Manhattan Bridge overpass." *Who's going to want to live in a place called Dumbo?* they figured, already sensing that their quiet, boho artists' colony might attract notice. Ultimately, it proved to be no deterrent. Not only did developers seize on Dumbo, it became the most expensive neighborhood in Brooklyn, with median home prices higher than such Manhattan neighborhoods as Greenwich Village and the Upper East Side. Old warehouses and lofts have been transformed into trendy residential and cultural venues. Luxury high-rises have been built on cobblestoned streets. And Dumbo has become a hub for creative types from muralists to furniture designers to filmmakers to tech entrepreneurs to culinary innovators. You'll see their influence on this walk, which also ventures into the tiny enclave of Vinegar Hill before wrapping up on the grounds of the Brooklyn Navy Yard.

Walk Description

Out of the subway, go to your right on York Street. At the end of the block on your right is a beloved factory building. Beloved for the glazed terra cotta ornamentation along the roofline, and beloved because of the treats that were made inside: Eskimo Pies. It's more identified with the ice cream pops (manufactured here from 1927 to 1966) than with the company that built it in 1909: Thomson Meter, whose monogram is on the corner shields at the top.

Turn left on Bridge Street.

Make a left on Front Street. The brick building on your right was erected in the early 1890s, when 65 shoe factories were operating in Brooklyn. This was the largest, Hanan & Son, whose retail locations extended to Europe and which employed more than 1,100 people at its peak (it went bankrupt in 1935). Down the block, Pedro's has been brightening this corner with its mural—and its margaritas—as long as anyone can remember. Its ramshackle appearance and inexpensive menu are welcome vestiges of a time before the neighborhood was even known as Dumbo.

Across Jay, the entire square block on the right was once occupied by the Grand Union super-market chain. From 1896 to 1915, it constructed six buildings here for a warehouse and a factory making teas, coffees, and spices. Visit the Shops at 145 Front, a collection of boutiques, art galleries, and designer showrooms. Of note to your left is Superfine, a Dumbo and foodie pioneer, having opened *way* back in 2001 with a focus on organic, sustainable ingredients.. It's in a building designed in 1888 by the Parfitt Brothers, prestigious architects of their day who are responsible for a number of Brooklyn's great Victorian-era residences and churches. Its original owner was E. W. Bliss, a major figure in Dumbo's industrial history: the machinery and sheet metal manufacturer, based in the area from 1870 to 1933, employed more than 1,600.

Walk under the Manhattan Bridge, then turn right on Adams Street. Visit the ❶ **PowerHouse Arena** on your left, where you'll find a bookstore, gift shop, and exhibition and performance space under one roof. The venue grew out of PowerHouse Books, a publishing company founded in Dumbo in 1995 that specializes in art and fashion books.

Turn left on Water Street. Those tracks going down Adams belonged to a rail system that transported goods within Gairville, as this district came to be known. When you reach Washington, look atop the brick building across to your right—a pediment with the Gair company's name is on the roof. It also shows two years: 1888, the year of the building's construction, and 1864, the year a Scottish immigrant named Robert Gair started manufacturing paper bags. He went on to invent machines to make corrugated paper and to fold boxes, and launched a cardboard-box factory that operated in this area from 1888 to 1927 with a workforce that reached 1,700—largest in the neighborhood.

A bunch of people are probably standing in the middle of the Washington–Water intersection taking pictures. Join them to behold an awesome view of the Empire State Building between the columns of the Manhattan Bridge.

Turn and walk away from the river on Washington. See Gair's name inscribed in the doorway on your left—this was the first of roughly 10 reinforced-concrete facilities he built. Another is to your right. Where did it fit in the company's chronology? He tells you at the corner with Front Street, along with the year of construction on the shield to the right above the door.

Turn right on Front, then make a right on Main Street. The Sweeney Building at #30 was a nickelware factory when it opened in 1911; now it's condos. Across Water Street on your left, the Stable Building was built by Gair for just that purpose in the 1880s and currently houses several art galleries. Check 'em out—some have entrances on Water.

On the other side of Main Street stands Dumbo's most recognizable landmark, the Clocktower Building. Completed in 1914, it was the final—and tallest—Gair building but now bears the name Walentas, after the developer who converted it to condos. Its triplex penthouse, which includes 14-foot clocks (you can see out of them) and a glass elevator, sold for $18 million in 2016. Walentas bought the whole building in the 1990s for a million.

From Main Street, go right on Plymouth Street—but look down Plymouth in the other direction at the Brooklyn Bridge, designed by John Roebling. Esteemed architecture critic Lewis Mumford once commented that the only person who had a bigger influence on the Brooklyn waterfront than Roebling was Robert Gair. At the Washington Street corner, visit the ❷ **Smack Mellon** gallery. In this building—an 1891 extension of Gair's first building that adjoins it—Smack Mellon has studios and production labs for artists in addition to its exhibition space. Across Plymouth, ascend the steps in Brooklyn Bridge Park to a terrace with stone slabs from which you can gain an even better view. The rest of this section of Brooklyn Bridge Park is covered in Walk 1 (see page 3).

From Plymouth, turn left on Adams Street. Bliss's factory occupied the entire block to your right.

Cross John Street and enter another section of Brooklyn Bridge Park via the path beside the new condo (which contains only 42 apartments, 4 of them penthouses). Follow the path to the left, crossing footbridges over a salt marsh and tidal channel. Look for the ziggurat-shaped metal relics arrayed in a sunken area with rocks. These were the footings of a demolished building of the Arbuckle Brothers' sugar refinery. A surviving structure from the refinery is now the other residential building on the park. As part of its recent conversion, the brick building is getting a new glass-and-steel facade on the water side—a look inspired by sugar crystals. Continue around that building and exit the park at Jay Street. The building to your right across Plymouth was erected in 1909 for the Arbuckles, following Robert Gair's lead regarding reinforced-concrete construction.

The Arbuckle Brothers employed 670-plus people in the sugar refinery, but their business actually revolved around coffee. They were pioneers in the packaging of roasted ground coffee—before their Ariosa brand was introduced, people had to roast their own coffee beans at home. The Arbuckles started producing sugar because they needed it as an ingredient in the glaze that was applied to the roasted coffee beans as a preservative. Their company grew into the world's largest coffee roaster and shipper, with its own fleet of vessels sailing to South America to get the raw materials.

On Jay Street at the left corner, in a building previously inhabited by the Arbuckles, ❸ **Brooklyn Roasting Company** has brought their discipline into the 21st century, roasting organic, fair-trade beans from places as far-flung as Bali, Peru, and Ethiopia in small batches—and also providing a spacious café–cum–reading room for customers.

Continuing up Jay, you next reach ❹ **GK Arts Center,** home to the ballet school and performing company run by Gelsey Kirkland, the onetime prima ballerina. Other dance and theater productions also take the stage in its 310-seat theater. At Plymouth Street, to the right are the art galleries A.I.R., which is dedicated to female artists, and Usagi, which contains a café serving Japanese teas and food.

Before turning left on Plymouth Street, look across the Jay–Plymouth intersection (to your right) to the redbrick building with an arched doorway on Jay. It was built in 1891 for Masury Paint, which patented the can with a thin pryable lid that we think of as a standard paint can. Masury's invention made it possible to sell ready-made paint, and the company maintained an exclusive patent on it for 21 years. Follow the old rail tracks from Jay to the left on Plymouth. #185, built for the Arbuckle Brothers in 1900, was used in the '40s and '50s for offices of Brillo (its scouring-pad factory was on John Street). The tall building at #195 was erected in 1892 as the metal spinning and plating plant of S. Sternau & Co., which invented a small burner called a Sternau—eventually spelled Sterno.

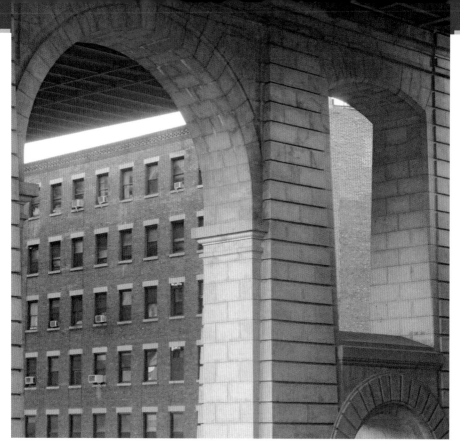

This is truly dumbo—down under the Manhattan Bridge overpass—on Pearl Street

Turn right on Bridge Street, as the rail tracks do. They go all the way into the lobby of the residential conversion at #37—originally built for Kirkman & Son's fat storage. They were soap makers, and the adjacent building was their glycerin plant. These were 1910s additions to their main facility across the street, #50, which was designed in 1894 by William Tubby, a leading residential architect of the late 19th century.

Turn left at Front Street, entering Vinegar Hill. The red garage door on the left is on a former firehouse, now a residence, built around 1855. #231–233 dates to 1908 and was designed by Tubby for a Benjamin Moore paint factory. It's followed by a row of Greek Revival brick townhouses. Most of them date to the 1840s; the second pair may have been built as early as the 1830s.

Vinegar Hill originated as a working-class community of Navy Yard employees and people who served as domestics in Brooklyn Heights. Today it's a 19th-century village scrunched between a power plant, a highway, and a housing project. Vinegar Hill's residents were predominately Irish throughout the 1800s, and local landowner John Jackson named it after a battle of Irish independence.

Turn left on Gold Street. These Greek Revival brick rowhouses on the right, including those at each end with street-level storefronts, are from the 1840s.

Turn right on Water Street. Go left at Hudson Avenue, then promptly right on Evans Street. At the end on your right is a gated property with a lawn and a pretty white mansion—looks more like a Hamptons estate than something you'd find in the city. This now privately owned house was built in 1806 for the Brooklyn Navy Yard commandant and designed by the same architect as the United States Capitol.

Go left on Little Street, which abuts the decommissioned but once mightily important Navy Yard. Shipbuilder John Jackson, who's considered the founder of Vinegar Hill, sold land to the US government in 1801 that was developed into the Navy Yard—which operated until 1966 and still has a few active dry docks (see page 140 for more about it). Vinegar Hill turned into a red-light district during the Navy Yard's tenure, earning the nickname Hell's Half Acre.

Turn left on Plymouth, then left on Hudson, the main drag of Vinegar Hill. Original ownership of both corner buildings has been traced to John Jackson's family: #49 may have been built as early as 1801. On the next block, Vinegar Hill House (#72) was the only retail business in the neighborhood when it opened in 2008—all these other storefronts were vacant or converted to residential. Opposite it, the three buildings between vacant lots have stood since 1817 and were originally Jackson property.

Continue on Hudson as it turns into Navy Street. A wonderful mural on your left illustrates neighborhood and Navy Yard history. Enter the Navy Yard after one more block, opposite Sands Street. Inside the gatehouse on your right is the tasting room of the **5 Kings County Distillery,** which has won awards for its bourbons, corn-based "moonshine," single-malt whiskey, and chocolate whiskey. The distillery itself is located inside the 1917 paymaster's building—straight ahead when you enter the Navy Yard grounds (tours are offered). From there, go to your right to the four-story building with a gazebo-type structure on its roof. Inside, ascend to **6 Rooftop Reds,** the world's first commercial urban rooftop vineyard—and also a delightful place to hang out. I mean, a hammock with this view . . . doesn't get much better than that! The vines grow in specially cultivated soil in custom-designed planters.

Go back on Navy to York, make a left, and return to the F train at Jay Street.

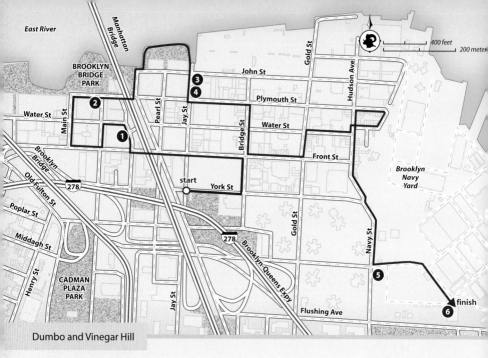

Dumbo and Vinegar Hill

Points of Interest

1. **Powerhouse Arena** 28 Adams St.; 718-666-3049, powerhousearena.com
2. **Smack Mellon** 92 Plymouth St.; 718-834-8761, smackmellon.org
3. **Brooklyn Roasting Company** 25 Jay St.; 718-514-2874, brooklynroasting.com
4. **GK Arts Center** 29 Jay St.; 212-600-0047, gkartscenter.org
5. **Kings County Distillery** Brooklyn Navy Yard gatehouse, 299 Sands St.; 347-689-4180, kingscountydistillery.com
6. **Rooftop Reds** Brooklyn Navy Yard, Building 275; 571-327-3578, rooftopreds.com

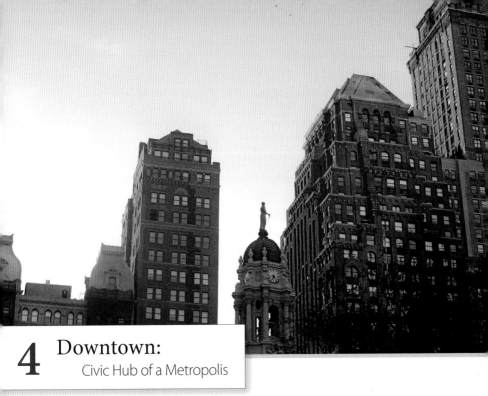

4 Downtown:
Civic Hub of a Metropolis

Above: Borough Hall (center) flanked by early skyscrapers on Court Street

BOUNDARIES: Johnson St., Flatbush Ave. Extension, State St., Clinton St.
DISTANCE: 2.5 miles
SUBWAY: A or C to Hoyt-Schermerhorn

Well, that only took a hundred years. . . . Brooklynites had anticipated a boom for Downtown Brooklyn when the then-independent municipality of Brooklyn was consolidated into the City of New York in 1898 as a borough. But instead of New York's business district spilling across the Brooklyn Bridge as expected, Manhattan expanded northward and Midtown developed as the new commercial center. But now, more than a century later, Downtown Brooklyn is finally getting its boom. Completed and planned construction is adding more than 10,000 apartments and nearly 1.5 million square feet of office space since 2004. Most hotel chains are opening properties in the neighborhood. And Brooklyn's three tallest buildings are all in Downtown, and all were completed since 2014. The real estate blog Bisnow summed up the goings-on in Downtown Brooklyn: "We're practically seeing a whole new city being built right before our eyes." There's still plenty left from the old city filling out Downtown's streetscape.

Walk Description

Upon exiting the subway, go to your right on Schermerhorn Street, then left on Hoyt Street. Turn right at State. The **❶ State Street Houses** comprise 23 residences in Greek Revival and Italianate styles that are recognized by both the city landmarks commission and the National Register of Historic Places. Most of them are on your left, #324–290, but they also include #299–291 on your right. They were not built as a unit but at different times between 1847 and 1874 and have been meticulously preserved—the cast-iron balconies outside #297–293 are original.

Before you turn right on Smith Street, look across to that tall building on the left. The dearth of windows may tip you off: it's the House of Detention—a jail whose presence has not deterred luxury residences from sprouting up en masse in the vicinity. Detainees are taken across State Street for their day in court, and you can check out the courthouse from different sides as you turn onto Smith and then left on Schermerhorn. Constructed during the Art Deco age but in an older Renaissance Revival style, this is the one elegant building among Downtown Brooklyn's otherwise plain courthouses. Those eagle-topped shields between the arches feature the seals of Brooklyn (on the left) and New York City (on the right) beneath the cherub faces. Farther down the block on Schermerhorn is the Friends Meeting House, used ever since it was built in 1857 for gatherings of Quakers, the religious society committed to peace and justice.

Make a right on Boerum Place. The building across the street, which has the address 22 Boerum Place on this side but officially is 110 Livingston Street, was designed by Beaux Arts icons McKim, Mead & White in 1926 for the Elks Club—with bowling alley, swimming pool, and guest rooms inside—but from 1939 to 2003 was the headquarters of the New York City Board of Education. The penthouse floors were added when it was converted to million-dollar condos.

Under the building, you find the **❷ New York Transit Museum,** located inside a deactivated subway station that you enter near the Schermerhorn corner. The museum's collection includes old buses, turnstiles, subway signage, trolley models, and vintage subway cars that visitors can board. At street level, 22 Boerum is home to ISSUE Project Room, an arts incubator that commissions and presents works in different performance genres.

Proceed north across Livingston Street, then take Red Hook Lane to your right. This alley is all that's left of a road that once extended to the neighborhood of Red Hook over a mile away—a road predating all development in Brooklyn, as it started as a Native American trail and was a strategic route during the American Revolution.

Turn right when you reach Fulton Street. Go inside #372 and seek out the mahogany bar, embossed walls, brass chandeliers, and cherrywood-framed mirrors. Gage & Tollner restaurant (specialty: clam bellies on toast) was responsible for the sumptuous Gay Nineties ambience—which, despite an interior landmarking, has dissipated as a series of eateries and shops have occupied the space since Gage & Tollner closed in 2004 after 112 years at this location. Continuing along Fulton, after Smith on your right there's a side entrance to the Brooklyn Tabernacle, whose gospel choir has won a Grammy Award.

This Fulton Mall was a lauded urban-renewal project in the 1970s and '80s but has been more controversial of late, as the increasingly affluent residents of surrounding neighborhoods complained about the strip's downscale character (decide for yourself if that's racially coded). While there are still plenty of street vendors and discount stores, a bunch of retail chains have opened along Fulton recently, and both the roadway and sidewalks have been renovated. Still the third-busiest shopping district in the city (after Manhattan's Herald Square and Madison Avenue), this section of Fulton Street was once *the* shopping destination of Brooklyn. Look up at the balconet wrapping around the corner building on your left across Lawrence Street. The entire site once belonged to women's clothier Oppenheim Collins—those are its initials entwined on the shield at the tippy-top.

On your right past Gallatin Place, ❸ **Macy's** fills two buildings facing Fulton: one from the 1870s with a cast-iron front and the other an Art Deco classic designed in 1929 by the architects of Saks Fifth Avenue and Bloomingdale's in Manhattan. Prior to 1995, these were A&S, which had anchored Fulton shopping ever since the street developed as a retail hub after the opening of the Brooklyn Bridge in 1883. The terra cotta flourishes on the beautiful white building at #420 include a bust that may or may not be Queen Victoria, the British monarch at the time of the building's construction in 1888. On the other side of Macy's, note the onion-domed turret and terra cotta urns along the top of the corner building.

Across Hoyt, the bronze work of the window bays and finials is the scene-stealer, and this 1920s building boasts charming iron balconies as well. This structure was the last addition to—and is the sole survivor of—a block of buildings occupied by Namm & Son, a prime competitor of A&S from the late 1800s into the 1950s. Both this building and the Offerman Building opposite it on Fulton have been landmarked. That building now occupied by Old Navy and Nordstrom Rack is still known to old-timers as Martin's, the department store here from 1922 to 1979. Built in the early 1890s, it is looking quite grand following a recent cleaning. Don't miss the lions at the

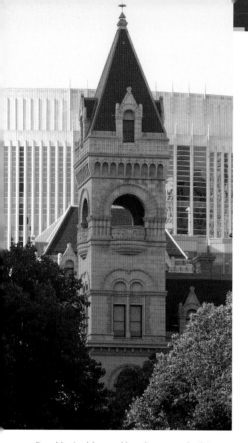

Brooklyn's old postal headquarters, built in the 1880s, with its new federal courthouse, opened in 2006, in the background

corners; the monogram beneath each is HO, for developer Henry Offerman.

On the east side of the Offerman Building, note that Duffield Street is also Abolitionist Place. This conaming resulted from an eminent-domain battle that ensued while this block of Duffield was being transformed over the past decade. The owner of the mid-19th-century house at #227 fought to save her home, as she believed it had been a stop on the Underground Railroad. The city's research could not conclusively establish that fugitive slaves had been sheltered there, but it conamed the street to commemorate all the antislavery activity that took place in the area. And 227 Duffield remains, surrounded by at least three new hotels. The owner hopes to open an abolition museum and heritage center inside.

Stay on Fulton past Duffield and then Elm Place, then go left onto the plaza, known as Albee Square. The name comes from the vaude-ville house built here in the 1920s by impresario Edward Albee. It was eventually converted to the RKO Albee movie palace, and shortly before the cinema was razed in 1977, it screened *Who's Afraid of Virginia Woolf?*, the film based on a play by Albee's namesake grandson. Now the mall that replaced the Albee theater has been demolished, too, supplanted by the brand-new mixed-use complex City Point, featuring stores, restaurants, the DeKalb Market food hall, and the first New York location of ❹ **Alamo Drafthouse Cinema**—a multiplex with service at your seat from a full menu and bar. It also has a macabre wax-museum-themed bar open to all.

There's an older structure on the north side of the plaza—the marble temple erected by the Dime Savings Bank in 1908. Its wonderful exterior detail includes carved bronze doors (the Brooklyn Bridge is one of the images) and a sculpture above the entry of two men along with symbols of agriculture and industry. The interior is fabulous, too: a rotunda of red marble columns with gilded capitals, inlaid with giant dimes. Thanks to air rights, this landmark, purchased by a developer in 2015, is slated to be incorporated into a skyscraper that would be Brooklyn's first over 1,000 feet tall. Facing the old bank, go to the left (on Fleet Street), then make a left on Flatbush Avenue Extension. Turn left on Willoughby Street, continuing around City Point's residential and office component.

Make a right on Duffield Street. Next to St. Boniface church are four pre-1850 houses that were relocated lest they be obliterated by Downtown's last megadevelopment, MetroTech, which was created in the 1990s. You're about to enter this 16-acre corridor encompassing office towers, a college campus, and public parkland.

At Myrtle Avenue, go left into ❺ **MetroTech,** whose office space is dominated by financial-services companies and government agencies. Watch on your left for a Tom Otterness sculpture in front of 2 MetroTech illustrating the local urban legend about alligators in the sewers. Look for more Otterness critters amid the lampposts to your right.

Walk across the Commons, a greensward with trees and seating, and then go to your right. You'll come to the NYU School of Engineering's Wunsch Hall, located in an 1846 church that housed Brooklyn's first black congregation, Bridge Street AWME, which still exists in Bedford-Stuyvesant. It was a station on the Underground Railroad and was visited by Harriet Tubman and Frederick Douglass.

Go to your right facing Wunsch, and take Bridge Street out of MetroTech. The Art Deco building on your left at Willoughby Street was constructed as the Long Island headquarters of New York Telephone and is now a condominium called BellTel Lofts. The building was designed by Ralph Walker, one of the country's preeminent Art Deco architects—and a favorite of the phone company in particular (he even designed Ma Bell's pavilion at the 1939 World's Fair).

Make a right on Willoughby, but do look again at the telephone building when you're across the street to appreciate its numerous setbacks. When you reach Lawrence Street, step back so you can take in the full Beaux Arts splendor of the 1898 structure on your right. But you also want to look at it closer up to see the objects depicted in stone around the door and the initials (TC) carved above—it is, in fact, a predecessor to the telephone company headquarters you just saw at Bridge Street. Next to it on Lawrence stands the 514-foot Brooklyner, which had a 2009–2013 reign as Brooklyn's tallest building; it's now No. 5.

Continue on Willoughby to Jay Street and turn right to see another former headquarters—that of the *city* of Brooklyn's fire department. You can't miss this terra cotta–adorned Romanesque Revival composition with two pyramidal roofs, the higher one atop a story fronted by a receding arch. It was built in 1892, when firefighters located fires by sighting them from the tower, then rushed to them via horse-drawn carriage—hence the broad entryway. After only six years, the building was demoted from department headquarters to plain ol' firehouse when Brooklyn became a borough of New York City.

Return to Willoughby, proceed west one more block to Pearl Street, and turn right. In 1867, Quakers started a school in the basement of their meetinghouse that you saw on Schermerhorn. In 1973 they moved into Brooklyn Law School's former building on your right. Doorway reliefs depict milestones in world legal history, including the Code of Hammurabi, Ten Commandments, Magna Carta, and United States Constitution. The building across the street has some impressive ornamentation of its own at the door and windows, populated with (mostly) mythological beings.

Turn left at the end of Pearl onto the pedestrian plaza. When you reach Adams Street, you're across from the State Supreme Court—a dowdy edifice that, surprisingly, was designed by the same firm that created the Empire State Building.

Make a left on Adams. In front of the Shake Shack at Fulton Street, cross Adams, putting you on Joralemon Street. Pause to look ahead to Court Street at the *old* skyline of Brooklyn: four buildings in a row that were successively the borough's tallest upon their completion between 1901 and 1927. Then make a right onto the path next to ❻ **Borough Hall.** Go all the way to the fountain, then turn around for your nice view of this exquisite Greek Revival structure, opened in 1849 as Brooklyn's City Hall.

Continue into the plaza, variously called Columbus Park or the Civic Center. To your right are two Kennedy memorials: a bust of Robert F. Kennedy, who represented New York State in the United States Senate, and a tree planted in memory of President John F. Kennedy. Next you greet Christopher Columbus. This famous sailor has moorings around the base of his pedestal.

As you continue to head north through the park, you can see the Manhattan Bridge off in the distance. The statue at this end is of Henry Ward Beecher, abolitionist pastor of nearby Plymouth Church (who usually wore a cape as shown). Beecher's advocacy for children and African Americans is represented in the figures at the base. The Romanesque fortress beyond Beecher is yet another headquarters demoted to branch when Brooklyn lost its city status; this one belonged to the Postal Service. The section facing Johnson Street—an extravaganza of dormers and turrets, with a potbellied arcade atop the tower—is the original structure, constructed from 1885 to 1891.

With the old post office to your right, walk on Johnson Street. Cross Cadman Plaza West and go left.

Make a right on Montague Street, stopping to read the plaque on the corner bank building. On the opposite corner with Court stands the tallest of the old skyscrapers you glimpsed from Adams Street. Completed in 1927, it was Brooklyn's first building with more than 30 stories.

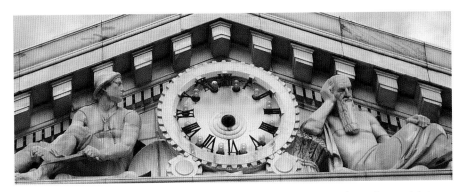

Morning and evening are symbolized by male figures at two different ages in the pediment of the former Dime bank on Albee Square

This block of Montague has remained "Bank Row," as it was a century ago, though the banks have new names. On your right, Citibank occupies a 1903 beaut designed by the same team as the Dime you saw near Fulton Street; the Art Deco skyscraper to its right (#185) was designed by architects who would next work on Rockefeller Center. At the corner of Clinton Street, Chase's 1915 building, modeled on a palace in Verona, Italy, features extraordinary ornamentation on its wrought-iron gates, entryway, and lampposts, as well as a gilded ceiling inside. Catercorner from Chase, the 1891 headquarters of the Franklin Trust Company has been converted to luxury apartments.

Turn left on Clinton Street, then left on Remsen Street. Past the church-turned-apartments on your right, St. Francis College took over a building erected in 1914 as headquarters of the gas company—thus the torches and gas lamps in the bronze ornamentation. The brownstone-and-brick #186 was created in the 1880s by the Parfitt Brothers, in-demand Brooklyn architects of the Victorian age. Next to it stands Brooklyn's tallest building from 1918 to 1926, when it was surpassed by the building on the opposite corner of Remsen and Court (which held the title only a year).

Turn right on Court Street. The Temple Bar Building at #44 was Brooklyn's tallest when opened in 1901—the oldest of these early skyscrapers. It's still a favorite of many, especially because of its cupolas. Stand right outside the door, facing the building, and look up for an interesting view.

At Joralemon, cross Court to your left to go to the subway—but wait, there's one last old skyscraper to see. Turning back toward Court, look to your left at the neo-Gothic "wedding cake" at the next corner (Livingston Street). Limestone and terra cotta take you from one setback to the next, with it all peaking in a cupola-crowned pyramidal roof.

Enter the subway on Joralemon in front of Borough Hall.

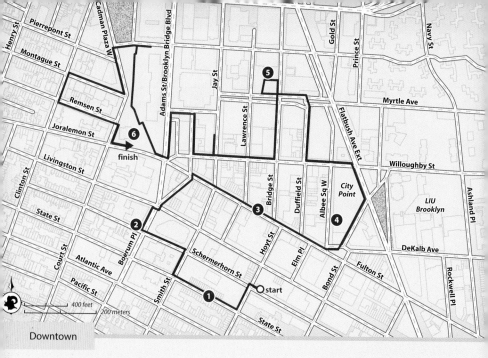

Points of Interest

1. **State Street Houses** 290–324 and 291–299 State St.

2. **New York Transit Museum** Boerum Place and Schermerhorn Street; 718-694-1600, nytransitmuseum.org

3. **Macy's** 422 Fulton St.; 718-875-7200, l.macys.com/brooklyn-downtown-in-brooklyn-ny

4. **Alamo Drafthouse Cinema and House of Wax** City Point, 445 Albee Square W.; 718-513-2547, drafthouse.com/nyc and 929-382-5403, thehouseofwax.com

5. **MetroTech** Myrtle Avenue and Bridge Street

6. **Borough Hall** 209 Joralemon St.; 718-802-3700, brooklyn-usa.org

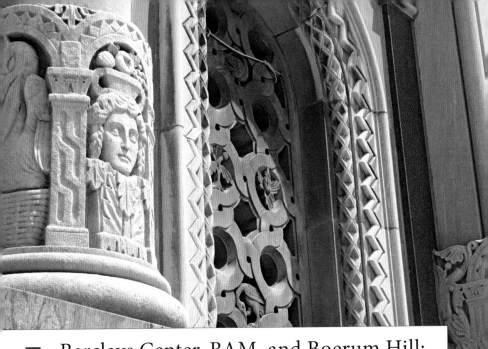

5 Barclays Center, BAM, and Boerum Hill:
Game On

BOUNDARIES: Lafayette Ave., Flatbush Ave., Wyckoff St., Boerum Pl.
DISTANCE: 2.3 miles
SUBWAY: B/D/N/Q/R/2/3/4/5 to Atlantic Ave./Barclays Center (Flatbush Ave./Atlantic Ave. exit)

Nothing will ever heal the wound of losing the Dodgers, but Brooklyn got back in the big leagues in 2012 when the Barclays Center opened and became the new home of the Nets, the NBA team previously based in New Jersey. The arena hosted the MTV Video Music Awards during its first year and is now a stop on many a pop star's world tour. It happens to be located just a couple of blocks from Brooklyn's *other* premier performance venue, the Brooklyn Academy of Music, known to all as BAM (pronounced as one syllable). Established in 1859 in Brooklyn Heights, BAM is the oldest performing arts institution in the country, yet it continues to expand and has spawned a cultural district around it. The arts presence—and high-rise construction—does not cease once you cross Flatbush Avenue into Boerum Hill. But the genteel residential streets of its historic district will take you back to another time, as they're full of classic mid-19th-century styles, with many homes predating the Civil War.

Walk Description

Come up the stairs from the subway and the ❶ **Barclays Center** is right in front of you. It resembles a spaceship, although those brown metal panels of the facade are meant to resemble Brooklyn's iconic brownstones. Walk straight ahead into the covered entry area that has a video-screen-ringed opening in the roof. Turn and walk through the plaza with planters and benches. Notice that both the arena's roof and the canopy of the subway station are covered with sedum plants—just one of the "green" components of this LEED-certified property. The first two performers to give concerts here, in the fall of 2012, were Brooklyn-born and -raised Jay-Z and Barbra Streisand. As of 2015, it's also home ice for the NHL's New York Islanders, who used to play in suburban Nassau County. Head to the flagpole at the Flatbush and Atlantic intersection; it has an important local pedigree, too, as you can learn from its plaque.

Cross Atlantic Avenue and walk on Flatbush Avenue beside the Atlantic Terminal mall. The subway station house on the island to your left dates to 1908, the year the subway first came to Brooklyn. Only three original control houses, as these structures are officially called, remain in the city, and this is the only one in Brooklyn.

At the corner of Hanson Place, stand before the ❷ **Williamsburgh Savings Bank** tower, aka One Hanson Place, and gaze up. For 80 years from the day it opened in 1929, this 512-foot domed clocktower stood as Brooklyn's only skyscraper—and then it was joined by a building only 2 feet taller (the Brooklyner on Lawrence Street). Today, alas, it ranks sixth, and at least four additional taller buildings have been proposed.

Cross Hanson Place and examine the detail on this magnificent building. Look for the lions guarding a lockbox, industrious folks depicted in the grille, griffins holding flagpoles. The former bank lobby, featuring marble floors and a zodiac-themed mosaic ceiling among other lavish trappings, has received its own interior landmark designation and has been the winter locale for the Brooklyn Flea and Smorgasburg markets.

Go to the building's Ashland Place side; at the base of the window columns, you find owls and pelicans alternating with human faces, while who knows what those creatures are peering between the paired arches. Many of the things sculpted on the exterior—beehives, squirrels with acorns—are symbols of thrift, ironic given what people are paying to live in the apartments inside. The building was converted to residential around 2007; in its commercial heyday, it had the nickname Tower of Pain because a lot of dentists had offices here.

Walk on Ashland Place. ❸ BAM is opening a venue inside the new 300 Ashland apartment building to your left. On your right is BAM Fisher, a 2012 addition containing a 250-seat theater, rehearsal space, and a rooftop terrace. Then you reach BAM's main building, and could anything be more welcoming than the musician cherubs around the doorways?

Go right on Lafayette Avenue to take in BAM in all its glory. This building, its home since 1908, boasts a 2,000-seat opera house whose ceiling is gilded like a Fabergé egg; a ballroom with 24-foot-high windows, now used as a cafe; and a multiscreen cinema. Tantamount to the physical splendor is BAM's artistic legacy—from one of Enrico Caruso's final performances to the annual Next Wave Festival.

With BAM on your left, walk west on Lafayette Avenue and you see BAM's cultural neighbors. First, at the corner of Ashland Place, look to your right at the dark gray building with a multistory windowed front: Theatre for a New Audience, a classical company that bounced around various locations in Manhattan and Brooklyn for 34 years before opening this building in 2013. Cross Ashland, passing the Mark Morris Dance Center, home of Morris's world-renowned company, but also a place for people of all ages and abilities to take dance and fitness classes.

Cross Flatbush Avenue and head toward the school and church buildings across the street from each other. But of course you can't miss the residential tower just beyond the church to your right: Hub, which topped out at 610 feet to become Brooklyn's tallest building in 2016.

Walk on 3rd Avenue between the school and church—or rather temple, constructed for Brooklyn's oldest Baptist congregation in 1893. Its interior was rebuilt after it was gutted by a fire in 1917, a disaster that occurred again in 2010. The school, meanwhile, was expanded multiple times from the 1890s and 1920s, but its oldest section dates to 1840, when it was built for a boys' boarding school. It was used as an infirmary during the Civil War. Across State Street, in the YMCA on your right, the 1920s Memorial Hall theater is the current home of arts organization ❹ Roulette, which was founded in downtown Manhattan in the '70s as an incubator of avant-garde musical composers and now presents music, dance, and multimedia performances.

Continue on 3rd to Pacific Street, where you can reminisce about the days when people not only read newspapers, but when a newspaper would invest in a building like the green-roofed one on your left, with long windows that allowed passersby to watch the printing, collating, and folding of papers. *The New York Times* built this printing plant (now a school) in the late 1920s, its marbleized exterior adorned with heads of royalty both human and leonine. Across the street stands Bethlehem Lutheran Church, whose name was preceded by "Swedish Evangelical" when this building was erected in 1894—during an era when Atlantic Avenue was known as Swedish Broadway.

Walk on Pacific past the church and then past playgrounds on both sides of the street.

Turn right at Nevins Street, then left on Atlantic Avenue, which slices east–west across the entire borough. The building on the right with arched windows, along with the building adjoining it to the left, was an Anheuser-Busch beer-bottling plant from the 1880s to 1903 and later became part of a factory complex that included the newer, taller building next to them. What else was manufactured there? It still says above the door on that taller building. Given the indelicate nature of the product, you may wonder why they didn't pry off the Ex-Lax name when the building went co-op. Well, at least they removed the words "The Ideal Laxative"!

Next you pass the House of the Lord, a Pentecostal church whose building was constructed for a Swedish church in the 1890s. On both sides of the avenue, Victorian storefronts and cast-iron street lamps preserve an old-fashioned ambience even as fashionable new retailers hang out their shingles. The corner on your right has been a church site since the 1850s—since 1957 for St. Cyril's of Turau, a Belarussian Orthodox church.

Cross Bond Street and you're in the midst of Antiques Row, or what's left of it. Atlantic Avenue had more than 30 antiques shops in the 1970s and '80s. Now it's down to a handful, mostly confined to the north (right) side of this block.

Turn left on Hoyt Street and peek into Hoyt Street Garden on the right. This oasis was created in 1975, when the area—like much of the then financially strapped city—was in shabby condition. The Presbyterian church next door owns the land but has given community volunteers complete control over the space. On your left, Mile End puts a Montreal-inspired spin on one of NYC's oldest cuisines, Jewish deli food—you can get your smoked brisket on top of poutine. The menu offers a "nibble" of the smoked meat in case you're not hungry enough for a sandwich or platter.

Turn left at Pacific Street. Past the nursing home on your right, the yellow-brick Cuyler Church, built in the 1890s, is now residential. In the 1930s and '40s its congregation included many Mohawk Indians, who had moved from Canada to New York City to work in skyscraper construction. The remainder of the block on that side consists of a variety of houses from either the early 1850s or early 1870s.

Turn right at Bond Street.

Make a right on Dean Street. The earliest homes here are the brownstone row about a third of the way down the block on the left side and the six brick rowhouses after it, all built between 1850 and 1852. On your right, the three houses closest to the nursing home also date to about 1850.

At Hoyt, the corner house across on your right was purchased by actors Heath Ledger and Michelle Williams in 2005; Ledger moved out shortly before his untimely death in January 2008. Turn left on Hoyt. The ➎ Brooklyn Inn, on your right at Bergen Street, may or may not be Brooklyn's oldest bar, but it's been open since 1885, which is when the fantastic exterior detail was added

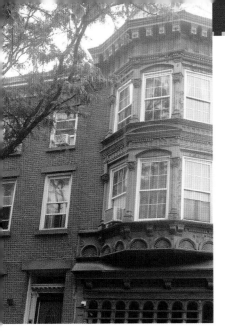
Dating to 1850, the Brooklyn Inn's building (right) on Hoyt Street was given a Queen Anne exterior in the 1880s

to this 1850 building. It was a brewery-owned saloon prior to 1919, a speakeasy during Prohibition, and had a restaurant on site briefly in the 1980s, but it's changed little inside—and the woodwork and stained glass are worth seeing.

Go left (east) on Bergen Street. The entire left side past the corner store–apartment building was built by one developer from 1869 to 1873. By that time, houses were being constructed in larger groups versus singly or just a couple at a time, as you've seen on other blocks.

Turn right on Bond and right again on Wyckoff Street. The first two houses after the community garden were erected in 1854 and set a no-stoop standard that was copied as more homes were built alongside them. Continue across Wyckoff to #108, whose facade, stoop, pavement, and even window bars are covered with a mosaic of tiles, beads, mirrors, and shells. And to think, it once probably looked just like its sedate next-door neighbor.

Turn right on Smith Street.

Make a left at Bergen Street. Drop in at ❻ **The Invisible Dog,** partway down on your right. This multidisciplinary arts center opened in 2009 in an ex-factory where the "invisible dog leash" novelty used to be manufactured. Encouraging collaboration and experimentation, the center contains artist studios, exhibition and performance space, and a pop-up store.

Turn right on Boerum Place, opposite a colorful row of Bergen Street clapboard houses, appearing impeccably maintained yet somewhat misplaced on this primarily commercial and brickfront block.

Go right on Dean Street. A couple of orphaned wood frame houses from the 1850s still stand toward the end of the block.

Turn right on Smith Street. Bar Tabac, at the right corner, was an early factor in Smith Street's reputation as a "restaurant row," and the French bistro has remained while many other restaurants on the street have come and gone.

The F/G subway station is at Bergen Street.

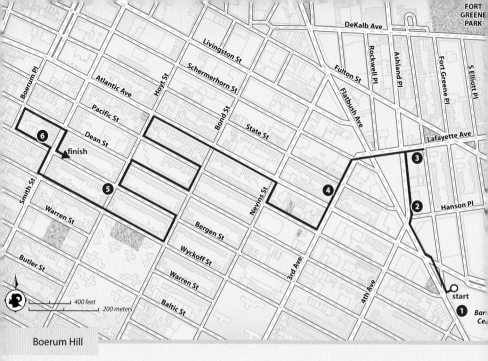

Boerum Hill

Points of Interest

1. **Barclays Center** 620 Atlantic Ave.; 917-618-6100, barclayscenter.com
2. **Williamsburgh Savings Bank clocktower** 1 Hanson Place
3. **Brooklyn Academy of Music** 30 Lafayette Ave.; 718-636-4100, bam.org
4. **Roulette** 38 3rd Ave.; 917-267-0363, roulette.org
5. **Brooklyn Inn** 148 Hoyt St.; 718-522-2525
6. **The Invisible Dog** 51 Bergen St., 347-560-3641, theinvisibledog.org

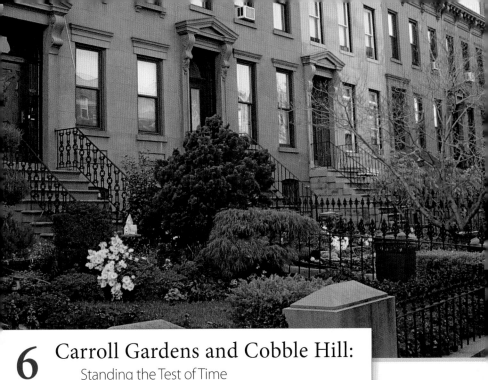

6 Carroll Gardens and Cobble Hill:
Standing the Test of Time

Above: *Within the Carroll Gardens Historic District, on Carroll Street*

BOUNDARIES: Atlantic Ave., Hoyt St., 2nd Pl., Hicks St.
DISTANCE: 2.9 miles
SUBWAY: F or G to Carroll St. (President St. exit)

The "Carroll" comes from Declaration of Independence signatory Charles Carroll; the "Gardens" from the unusually large plots of land bestowed on each house in an 1846 design for the neighborhood conceived by surveyor Richard Butts. Those deep front yards were well cared for over the years by garden-loving Italians, who moved to the area for the longshoreman work and were the dominant immigrant group here throughout the 20th century. Today most parts of Carroll Gardens are unrecognizable as a working-class community, as its proximity to Manhattan and abundance of brownstones have attracted an upscale populace. Cobble Hill, which borders Carroll Gardens to the north, first emerged as a fashionable residential district in the mid–19th century. A plethora of specialty shops and dining destinations that opened over the past 15 years have added a new facet to these neighborhoods rich in historic homes and churches along tree-lined streets.

Walk Description

Exit the subway at Smith and President Streets, and head west on President beside ❶ **Carroll Park.** Use the second entrance to the park, opposite a row of brownstones. Walk straight ahead to the memorial for local World War I casualties. Note that the surnames of the fallen are primarily Irish, Scandinavian, and East European; by World War II, the area's Italian population would surge. One indicator of the Italian influence in the neighborhood lies nearby: the bocce alley alongside one edge of the basketball courts. Go to your left, passing between playgrounds and to the left of the parkhouse, and exit down the steps onto Smith Street.

Cross Smith and walk straight onto President Street. You're now within Carroll Gardens' small historic district, developed entirely between 1869 and 1884.

Turn right on Hoyt Street. Those first four brick rowhouses on your left are the oldest homes in the historic district.

Turn right on Carroll Street. All the houses on this block date from 1871–74, except for #297 and #299, which were built in 1986 to fill a gap left after a former Norwegian church burned down.

Turn left on Smith Street. When the Gowanus Canal—located on the other side of Hoyt—was thriving as a commercial waterway in the first half of the 20th century, this was a strip of taverns and rooming houses for laborers.

Turn right on 2nd Place. To your left is a community garden on MTA-owned land.

Turn right on Court Street, then left on 1st Place.

Make a right at Clinton Street, across from an 1856 church that has been converted from Westminster Presbyterian to the Norwegian Seamen's Church to apartments. At the next corner on your left, the F. G. Guido Funeral Home occupies an 1840 mansion that's considered one of the city's finest examples of Greek Revival architecture. Diagonally across the Carroll Street intersection stands St. Paul's Episcopal. Its architect was one of its parishioners, Richard M. Upjohn, a Gothic master like his father, Richard Upjohn.

Make a right on President, where you pass a variety of freestanding residences and apartment houses before returning to brownstone uniformity. The magnificent 1893 home at #255 used to be the rectory of South Congregational Church—hence, the churchlike windows on the top level. Next to it, the church's ladies parlor (1889) has also become a private home, while the 1850s church itself was turned into an apartment co-op in the early 1980s. Take note of the twisted-rope shape of the property's lampposts, an homage to the neighborhood's maritime ties.

Turn left on Court Street, where G. Esposito, Monteleone's, and Marco Polo preserve the traditional Italian flavor on a block also home to newer businesses like a yoga studio and fro-yo joint. And what could better represent the upscaling of the neighborhood than the big new residential complex on your left past Union Street? On the right, the ❷ Brooklyn Strategist offers drop-in board-game playing. They have more than 500 games to choose from—not one involves a computer or smartphone. Continuing along the street, you pass some longstanding Italian food purveyors. You also pass from Carroll Gardens into Cobble Hill, but does that happen at Sackett or at Degraw Street? There are no official borders, and some people may say it's at another street.

Turn left at Kane Street. The ❸ Kane Street Synagogue on your left is the "Mother Synagogue of Brooklyn," home to its oldest Jewish congregation. Built in 1856 as a Dutch Reformed church, it's been a synagogue since 1905. Aaron Copland was bar mitzvahed here—and was encouraged to pursue his interest in music by the rabbi, Israel Goldfarb, a liturgical composer.

Make a left on Tompkins Place, a one-block street of 1840s and 1850s classics that you could enjoy for their door enframements alone.

Turn right on Degraw and then head back to Kane via another one-blocker, Strong Place. At the corner with Degraw is a recent church-to-condo conversion. This 1852 building, designed by Minard Lafever, a preeminent church architect of the time, had stood vacant and neglected for nearly a decade before being acquired by the condo developer.

Turn right at Kane, walking beside Christ Church, the oldest Episcopal church building in Brooklyn. Come around to its front on Clinton Street, and stand beneath the 120-foot, four-spire steeple. This 1842 masterpiece was designed by Richard Upjohn and was completed while his most famous project, Trinity Church at the head of Wall Street in Manhattan, was under construction. Christ Church's altar, pulpit, and some windows were designed by Louis Comfort Tiffany.

Go in the other direction on Clinton. On your left across Baltic Street, #296 was the home of Richard Upjohn, who also designed it (in 1842), although with only three stories (another was added later) and with a bay window rather than the slightly thrust front that replaced it.

Walk west along Baltic Street next to the Upjohn house. Richard M. Upjohn designed this apartment-house extension to his father's former home in 1893. Farther down on the right is the neighborhood's oldest long row of houses built together, starting with #181 and extending to the end of the block. They've all been modified one way or another since they were erected in 1837–39.

On the next block, you need only peek into the mews next to 145 Baltic, as you'll be going into it shortly, but look for the plaque on the side of 141 Baltic that tells you its name: COTTAGES

FOR WORKINGMEN. Hmm. In the meantime, don't overlook the handsome twin houses on both sides of Warren Place. Finishing out the block, you have the Home and Tower buildings to your left and right, respectively, which today constitute the Cobble Hill Towers.

At Hicks Street, first go left and check out the Home apartments, as they were known when they went up in the late 1870s in tandem with the Tower across Baltic. Both were built for the working class—"model tenements," offering those of modest means attractively designed housing with decent plumbing and ventilation. Then turn around and walk north on Hicks in front of the Tower complex.

Turn right on Warren Street, then enter ❹ **Warren Place** on your right. This was another development for the working class created by Alfred Tredway White, the altruistic businessman also responsible for Tower and Home, who'd been enlightened about London's experiments in upgraded worker housing by the newspaper reports of local journalist Walt Whitman. Today, of course, even these narrow abodes are affordable only to those with incomes far above workingmen's, as their privacy, splendid foliage, and backyards are uncommon luxuries in New York City. Take one path through Warren Place when you enter and the other on your way out. Then continue to the right on Warren Street.

Cobble Hill Park

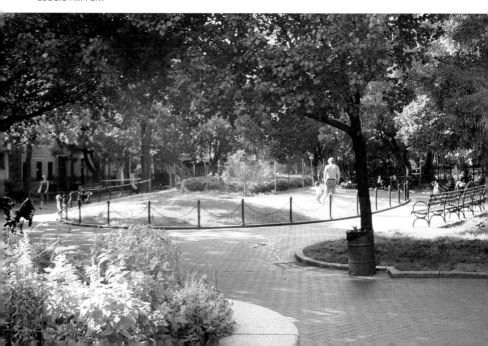

Turn left on Henry Street. The entire west side of the block is occupied by Cobble Hill Health Center, now a nursing home but built as a church-affiliated charity hospital in 1888.

Turn right on Verandah Place, which was probably an alley of stables and carriage houses before the houses were built in the 1850s. Thomas Wolfe lived in the basement of #40 in 1930 and described it in *You Can't Go Home Again:* "follow the two-foot strip of broken concrete pavement that skirts the alley, and go to the very last shabby house down by the end. . . . The place may seem to you more like a dungeon than a room that a man would voluntarily elect to live in." Don't despair—he also wrote that "he found beauty" here, from "a tree that leaned over into the narrow alley . . . ."

Turn left on Clinton Street and enter ❺ **Cobble Hill Park**—which may look like it's always belonged in this neighborhood but is a fairly recent addition. After a 100-year-old church on the spot was torn down around 1960 to make way for a supermarket, local residents rose up in opposition and were able to get the plans changed to a park. Go to the right in the park and come out on Congress Street and head to the left.

Turn right again at Henry. On your left as you approach Amity Street is a regal structure built for those in need. Toward the top it bears the name THE POLHEMUS CLINIC, founded in 1895 to provide medical services for poor residents of the waterfront district (the harbor's just two blocks beyond). Long Island College Hospital, of which Polhemus was part, closed in 2014, and now its entire site is targeted for mixed-use redevelopment.

Turn right on Amity. The busily embellished corner building on your right was also part of the hospital, opened as a nurses' dormitory in 1902. Upon crossing Clinton, notice the corner house on the right that is considered Cobble Hill's prize property, partly because of its generous yard. Known as the Degraw mansion, the house was built in 1845 in the simple Greek Revival mode— still evident from the first three stories of windows facing Clinton (the low iron fence is original, too). Without a lot of other buildings in the way at that time, it had a view of the water. The house was extended down Amity in an 1890 remodeling that also gave it the Flemish gable and large brownstone stoop. Down Amity on your left, #197 was the birthplace in January 1854 of Miss Jeanette Jerome, later known as Jennie Churchill, the American-socialite mother of Winston.

Turn left on Court Street. On the left at Atlantic Avenue, the first Brooklyn ❻ **Trader Joe's** is in a 1922 bank building whose outstanding features include cornice eagles and a high embossed ceiling. Read the plaque to the right of the door about the American Revolution fort on this site. This is also where a hill identified on a 1760s map as Cobleshill was located; after the name was rediscovered in the 1950s, it was adapted for the neighborhood, which until then had just been considered an outpost of Brooklyn Heights or Red Hook.

Continue north on Court Street four blocks to reach the Borough Hall subway station.

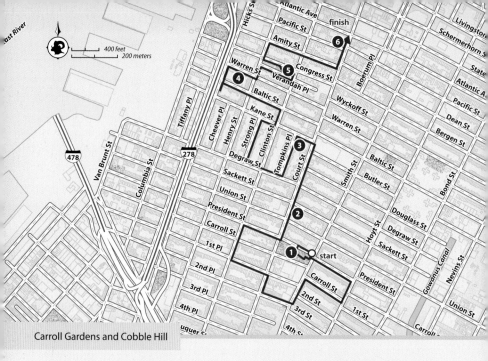

Carroll Gardens and Cobble Hill

Points of Interest

1 **Carroll Park** Smith and President Streets; nycgovparks.org

2 **The Brooklyn Strategist** 333 Court St.; 718-576-3035, thebrooklynstrategist.com

3 **Kane Street Synagogue** 236 Kane St.; 718-875-1550, kanestreet.org

4 **Warren Place Cottages for Workingmen** off Warren Street east of Hicks Street

5 **Cobble Hill Park** Clinton and Congress Streets; nycgovparks.org

6 **Trader Joe's (originally South Brooklyn Savings Institution)** 130 Court St.; 718-246-8460, traderjoes.com

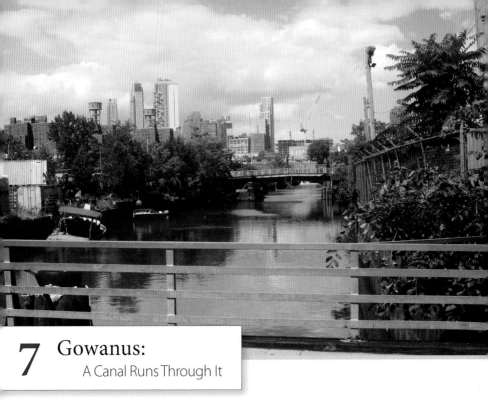

7 Gowanus:
A Canal Runs Through It

Above: Brooklyn's new residential towers and the Union Street bridge over the Gowanus Canal are part of the northern view from the historic Carroll Street Bridge

BOUNDARIES: Degraw St., 5th Ave., 9th St., Smith St.
DISTANCE: 3.1 miles
SUBWAY: F or G to Smith–9th St.

Superfund, what Superfund? In 2010 the EPA smacked the Gowanus Canal, once the nation's busiest commercial canal, with that designation signifying optimal toxicity. You might have expected it to dissuade construction of fancy apartments on its shores or an influx of commercial enterprises to the area, but instead, more and more people kept coming to Gowanus, the neighborhood around the canal. Some came here to live, new residents relocating from pricier brownstone neighborhoods nearby or drawn to the emerging arts community; others were just visitors who'd heard about that great new clam bar or Korean barbecue or alternative arts space or archery center or some other quirky establishment that had opened to much buzz. By the time the Superfund cleanup was set to begin in 2017, Gowanus had been dubbed the hottest neighborhood in Brooklyn. Its gritty character has not disappeared entirely, however, in part because it still has an active industrial sector.

Walk Description

You disembark at the highest elevated-train station in the world. The Culver viaduct was built 90 feet high to clear tall-masted ship traffic on the Gowanus Canal. Down on the street, you see a mix of residential and commercial, old and new typical of Gowanus . . . although some people will tell you you're actually in Red Hook or Carroll Gardens. You may also recognize this spot from a scene between Robert De Niro and Lorraine Bracco in *GoodFellas*.

Walk east on 9th Street, going under the viaduct and over the canal. Enter the Gowanus Industrial Arts Complex on your left, where old factories and warehouses are occupied by designers, craftspeople, and small manufacturers. You may be able to visit some—just follow the signs. Or simply enjoy the, er, scenic lookout. You can watch the train you were just on coming around a bend.

The 1.8-mile Gowanus Canal was created in the 1840s when a natural creek was extended for mercantile access to the bay, and cargo transporters relied on it for about a century. At the same time, it was collecting toxins from local foundries, gas plants, paint manufacturers, and the like. After the Gowanus Expressway (visible to your left) rendered the canal obsolete, it was left to fester for decades. So that's how we got to Superfund status—although the city and state had already undertaken a cleanup that was flushing the canal regularly with freshwater and had made it more or less tolerable fragrance-wise.

Return to 9th Street and continue in the same direction, passing other studios, showrooms, and stores.

Turn left on 2nd Avenue.

Make a right on 7th Street. This may seem like a remote, desolate location, but it doesn't keep indie-rock fans from flocking here for concerts at ❶ **The Bell House.** Music's not all that goes on in this former printing plant; it also hosts podcast tapings, comedy shows, dance parties, quiz nights, readings, and other events. On this same block, the rehabbed building at #168 holds art, design, and music studios.

Turn right on 3rd Avenue. Some of the creativity coming out of Gowanus is edible—such as ❷ **Four & Twenty Blackbirds** pie makers par excellence, on your left as you reach 8th Street.

Go left at 9th Street. The American Legion hall on the left is a converted church that was fashioned out of a pair of rowhouses. It was a meaningful location for the veterans group: what's now the 9th and 3rd intersection was the original burial ground for casualties of the Maryland 400 regiment, who played a strategic role in the Battle of Brooklyn.

At 4th Avenue, dramatic buildings stand at three of the four corners. Above the convenience store on the left, look up at the brickwork and additional (weathered) embellishment on the top floors—also see the lovely sculpting beneath the lower windows on the avenue side. Massive St. Aquinas church is in fine condition for its 130-plus years. Good Shepherd's building opposite it dates to 1876, when it was constructed for a Democratic clubhouse. A row of charming bay-windowed houses is also on that side of 9th Street, but the building you really want to watch for is on the left, current home of Slope Music school. This photogenic 1856 Second Empire villa features iron-crested end pavilions and a cupola. The family that built it lived here only five years; later it would serve as the offices of Higgins Ink, whose 8th Street brick factory you can see behind the house.

Turn left on 5th Avenue, a commercial street of Park Slope (whether the Slope–Gowanus border is 4th or 5th Avenue is a matter of debate) that was predominantly Latino and working-class into the 2000s. Evidence of that may still exist, but it's getting crowded out by higher-end new shops and eateries. Some of them sell unique merchandise. Where else, for instance, can you buy X-ray glasses, canned antimatter, and a secret-identity kit besides the Brooklyn Superhero Supply Co., on your left between 6th and 5th Streets? All sales benefit a youth writing program.

The middle school on the next block is named for the commander of the Maryland 400, General William Alexander, aka Lord Stirling. Past that, enter Washington Park and proceed to the ❸ Old Stone House, a 1930s replica of the Dutch farmhouse that had been constructed about a hundred feet to the east in 1699. It was at that house in the middle of the night on August 27, 1776, that a volunteer regiment of 400 Marylanders engaged a much larger force of British and Hessian soldiers in a battle—a tactical maneuver to allow the Continental Army to evacuate Brooklyn. The diversion succeeded, but nearly 300 of the Maryland men were killed. A small Battle of Brooklyn museum is inside the Old Stone House. As if that's not enough history, these grounds would become the first home field, from 1883 to 1891, of the baseball team eventually known as the Brooklyn Dodgers.

Today, in addition to celebrating its Revolutionary, sports, and agricultural heritage, the Old Stone House presents musical and theater performances, crafts and fitness classes, children's activities, and other cultural and social events.

Exit the park on 3rd Street and go left. As you near 3rd Avenue, the Old American Can Factory is on your left. This complex of six adjoining buildings constructed between 1865 and 1901 is yet another home for artists and creative businesses. These tenants are "curated"—interviewed and specially selected by the landlord. How about the artistry *outside*? The corner building especially is striking, with diamond-shaped windows facing 3rd Avenue.

Go to the right on 3rd Avenue but only as far as the whitish wall on your right. This is a remnant of the outfield wall of the second Washington Park, built for the Dodgers in 1898 by their new owner, Charles Ebbets, who'd started working for the club as a ticket taker. The Dodgers played at this park until they moved to Ebbets Field in 1913.

Turn and head back to 3rd Street, this time focusing on the ❹ **Whole Foods** corner, a spot that epitomizes Gowanus's transformation. Right through 2012, this entire block was just an empty lot except for that corner palazzo, which was vacant and dilapidated—its brick refacing chipping away, steps crumbling, columns covered with graffiti, windows boarded up. Whole Foods paid for the refurbishment of this landmark, believed to be New York City's earliest concrete building. It was erected in 1872–73 for the company that made the concrete, Coignet Stone, which also supplied concrete for St. Patrick's Cathedral, among other future landmarks.

Go inside the huge Whole Foods, which includes a beer growler fill-up, a sushi and ramen station, a voluminous salad bar, and a bakery that carries goods from Brooklyn-based purveyors. Go up to the roof deck, where there's a commercial greenhouse, children's playroom, bar with craft beers on tap (and a happy hour), table seating, and, of course, views!

Back downstairs, follow the esplanade alongside the canal from the south side of the store to 3rd Street. That large redbrick building you see with tall arched windows—and possibly graffiti—is an abandoned 19th-century rail power station, nicknamed the Batcave, and due to be renovated for arts purposes. Take the 3rd Street bridge over the canal.

Turn right on Bond Street, where a number of upscale residential projects intersperse with traditional housing. Go right on 2nd Street for access to the brand-new public waterfront park created in conjunction with the new canal-side apartment buildings. It includes a new launch for the ❺ **Gowanus Dredgers,** which offers canoes and kayaks for free public use on weekends— and has been doing so since 1999, so they must get credit for early advocacy of restoring the canal for recreational use (and environmental benefits). Follow the park's path to Carroll Street and go right. Walk the wood planks of the oldest retractile bridge in the United States, noting the track mechanism to your right used to "roll" the 1889 bridge open.

Turn left on Nevins Street. The Crusader Candle Co. to your right works with doors open in warmer weather, as the scent may indicate. At the next corner, pause to look at the old National Packing Box Factory across Union Street, another former industrial site given over to art and design space, including a pottery showroom at the ground-level corner.

Go right on Union Street. The ice cream emporium Ample Hills, on the right, has a rooftop patio. Their menu of creative concoctions includes It Came From Gowanus—dark chocolate ice cream stuffed with pieces of cookie, brownie, and white chocolate so as to resemble, but

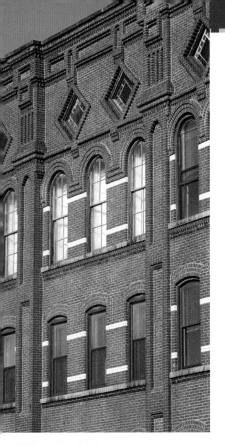

Old American Can Factory

obviously not taste like, toxic sludge. If you'd like to further feel as if you're at a summer resort, drop in a few doors down at Royal Palms Shuffleboard Club, boasting 10 courts plus bars serving up tropical cocktails.

Turn right on 3rd Avenue. When Gowanus was populated by longshoremen and other blue-collar types, they were predominantly Italian, and their imprint has not eroded completely. Witness, to your left, the red-sauce joint Two Toms, in business since the '40s under the same family's ownership, and on your right past President Street, the Glory Social Club, a "no girls allowed" hangout for *paisans* that's been around since 1927.

Make a left on Carroll Street. The wide-arch-windowed building on your left is a former bakery, constructed in the 1890s, that's been renovated for "boutique manufacturing" and other tenants. On your right, past the front doors of Our Lady of Peace Church, note all the Italian surnames in the World War II memorial.

Turn left on 4th Avenue. On your right after you cross President, a Blink gym occupies the circa-1907 Public Bath No. 7, decorated with seashells, fish, and tridents in polychromatic terra cotta. As you continue north, colorful civic-themed murals cover a few buildings.

Turn left on Degraw Street, and at the end of the block go into ❻ **Brooklyn Boulders,** a rock-climbing mecca inside a former garage for *Daily News* delivery trucks. Doesn't matter if you'd never try the sport, you've *got* to see this amazing facility with a variety of brightly painted climbing walls, murals, a café, dance studio, and weight room.

Return to 4th Avenue at Union for the R train. If you want to wrap up your time in Gowanus by sampling local craft beers, Threes Brewing is on Douglass (the next street north of Degraw) and Strong Rope Brewery is on President, both of them just off 4th Avenue on this side.

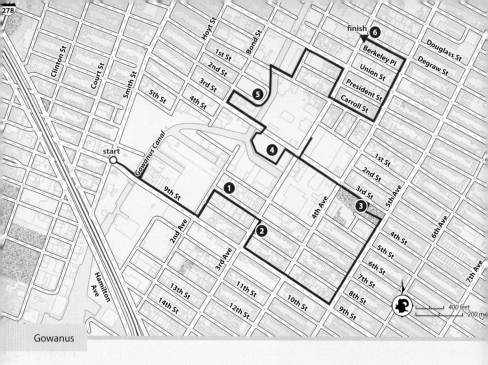

Gowanus

Points of Interest

1. **The Bell House** 149 7th St.; 718-643-6510, thebellhouseny.com
2. **Four & Twenty Blackbirds** 439 3rd Ave.; 718-499-2917, birdsblack.com
3. **Old Stone House** Washington Park, 336 3rd St.; 718-768-3195, theoldstonehouse.org
4. **Whole Foods** 214 3rd St.; 718-907-3622, wholefoodsmarket.com/stores/thirdand3rd
5. **Gowanus Dredgers** 2nd Street at the Gowanus Canal; 718-243-0849, gowanuscanal.org
6. **Brooklyn Boulders** 575 Degraw St.; 347-834-9066, brooklynboulders.com

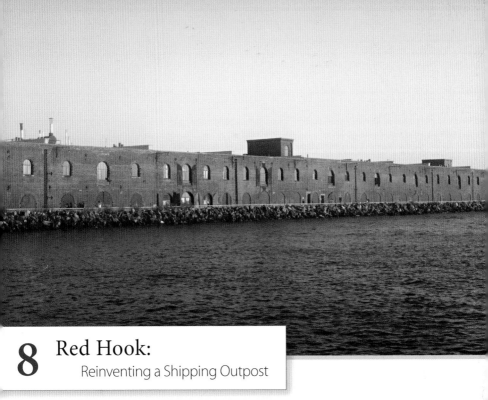

8 Red Hook:
Reinventing a Shipping Outpost

Above: At the foot of Van Brunt Street, Civil War–era warehouses extend onto the pier

BOUNDARIES: Seabring St., Otsego St., Erie Basin Park, Valentino Pier
DISTANCE: 3.4 miles
SUBWAY: A, C, G to Hoyt-Schermerhorn or 2, 3 to Hoyt St.; transfer one block west on Smith St. to B61 bus to Windsor Terrace

When the bus turns onto Van Brunt Street from Hamilton Avenue, you see the Red Hook Terminal in front of you. This is what remains of the commercial shipping industry that drove Red Hook's economy and shaped life in the community for generations. Between a drop-off in the shipping trade and construction of the Gowanus Expressway (which basically cut the peninsula off from the rest of Brooklyn), Red Hook grew isolated and dicey as the 20th century wore on. It had begun to gentrify when Hurricane Sandy hit in 2012, causing extensive damage. Since then, Red Hook has emerged as an epicurean destination thanks to a variety of restaurants as well as distilleries, chocolatiers, and other food and drink producers that serve their fare right where it's made. There's no denying the fun and funky artistic vibe that continues to spread through the neighborhood. Yet somehow Red Hook's coarse past—it's the place that launched Al Capone's career and inspired such hardscrabble tales as *Last Exit to Brooklyn,* Arthur Miller's *A View from the Bridge,* and *On the Waterfront*—is part of the charm, too.

Walk Description

Get off the bus on Van Brunt at Commerce Street and walk back one block to Seabring Street. Have a look at the former firehouse fronting Van Brunt at the far corner. Its right and left halves are identical (signage for current tenants notwithstanding)—a double house built in 1872 for a ladder company and an engine company.

Go onto Seabring Street. A couple of doors in on your left, visit ❶ **Raaka Virgin Chocolate.** "Virgin" refers to the organic, unroasted beans used to make high-percentage-cacao (very dark) bars in such flavors as bourbon-cask-aged, ghost pepper, and smoked chai. Near the end of this industrial block, watch for the "Greetings from . . . Red Hook" mural on the right.

Turn right on Richards Street, noting the honorary sign above you designating this Seven In Heaven Way. The seven firefighters from the station across the street who died at the World Trade Center had arrived on the scene before the second tower was hit.

Turn right on Commerce Street and proceed across Van Brunt. The huge buildings flanking Commerce on Imlay Street were erected around 1912 for the New York Dock Co., which owned a vast network of piers, factories, rail terminals, boats, and warehouses such as these in service of the Atlantic Basin, a port facility (behind the buildings) that was in operation for some 150 years. 160 Imlay has been converted to luxury condos.

Turn left and walk on Imlay to Pioneer Street. Right in front of you is ❷ **Pioneer Works,** which quickly became a social and artistic hub of the neighborhood following its 2012 opening. Practitioners of various arts, music, and sciences create and collaborate inside the vast former warehouse. You are welcome to visit its exhibitions and artist-in-residence studios, and to enjoy the delightful adjacent garden.

Diagonally across from the garden, enter the parking lot at the gate labeled PORTSIDE and head over to the red tanker docked there. It's the *Mary A. Whalen,* now maintained by the harbor education, advocacy, and preservation organization ❸ **PortSide NewYork** and one of the few remaining intact motorized coastal tankers of her era.

Out of the lot, walk east on Pioneer, crossing Van Brunt. On your right, #111 was built in 1878 as the Norwegian Seaman's Church. Today it's known as the Robotic Church, studio of Amorphic

Robot Works, which makes computer-controlled pneumatic sculptures. Fifty of their mechanized skeletons give scheduled "performances" inside. You may still see the name of a prior inhabitant on the building, Smo~King, a manufacturer of ashtrays and barbecues.

At Richards Street, go into Coffey Park. Near the flagpole, turn back toward Richards and the Visitation of the Blessed Virgin Mary's belltower. Try to see the interior of this Gothic church, featuring Italian frescoes, Tiffany windows, and a wooden ceiling shaped like a boat's keel—appropriate for a parish originally composed of Italian and Irish dockworkers.

Those buildings looming off to the east and south of the park are the Red Hook Houses, where more than half the neighborhood's residents live. One of the oldest and largest public housing projects in the city, it opened during the Depression for dockworkers and their families but gained notoriety in the late 20th century as drugs and crime ran rampant.

Stroll through Coffey Park, then exit on Richards at Visitation Place (between Pioneer and Verona) and go straight. The Red Hook Community Justice Center on your right, opened in 2000, is a nationwide model for criminal-justice reform, focusing on mediation and alternatives to incarceration like training, treatment, and community service.

Make a left on Van Brunt, Red Hook's main commercial street. Notice the doughboy statue to your left past King Street, then pop into an art gallery, bar, or boutique. The block of Van Brunt past Wolcott Street is full of Red Hook stalwarts—which is to say, older than 10 years—on your left, including the ❹ **Kentler International Drawing Space,** a true pioneer of Red Hook's arts community. It's been showcasing contemporary works on paper since 1990, and took its name from the original building owner (see up top).

Turn right on Dikeman Street.

Make a left on cobblestone Conover Street. The building on the right that says ❺ **Cacao Prieto** houses both the chocolatier of that name and Widow Jane Distillery, also owned by Mr. Prieto Preston. His family's farm in the Dominican Republic supplies all the cacao beans, which are used to make chocolate bars infused with such flavors as absinthe, bergamot, and spice, as well as a line of liqueurs and rums. You can shop, taste, and tour both the whiskey and chocolate enterprises. Plus, there's an inner courtyard where peafowl roam amid patio furniture.

Turn right on Coffey Street, looking up on your right at the engraved PARTITION STREET on the corner building. The street was rechristened in the early 1900s in honor of Michael Joseph Coffey, a politician who served the area for over 30 years. The fine brick homes on this block were built in the 1800s. No one knows for sure exactly what took place around here in 1776, but it's believed George Washington's troops fled the British onslaught during the Battle of Long Island through marshlands that are now Red Hook—hence the RED HOOK LANE HERITAGE TRAIL street signs posted in places.

Look both ways at Ferris: between the Belgian-block paving (colloquially called cobblestone) and aging industrial structures, this street evokes the Red Hook of yore. The site to your right, however, had been earmarked for the Red Hook of tomorrow: the Red Hook Innovation Studios, a campus of offices and workspace for creative industries (like design and tech) that would include a waterfront promenade and a park. This 19th-century brick warehouse at the corner would be renovated into an event venue within the complex. The project had yet to advance past planning stages at press time.

You'll probably catch a glimpse of the Statue of Liberty before you reach the entrance to Valentino Pier near the end of Coffey Street. Popular for fishing and sunset gazing, this spot is the closest you can get to Lady Liberty on land, and benches and a beach contribute to its overall pleasantness. The pier is now accepted as the site of Fort Defiance, a Revolutionary War post destroyed by the British, though its precise location is not known. Looking to your left, the venue at the tip of Pier 41 with floor-length windows is Liberty Warehouse, where Jay-Z held the release party for his 2013 album *Magna Carta Holy Grail*.

Leaving the pier, go to your right at the flagpole onto the path leading between brick warehouses. A 1953 Ford is parked in front of Steve's Authentic Key Lime Pies, where you can refresh with a Swingle chocolate-coated frozen pie on a stick.

With your back to Steve's, go to your right and onto Van Dyke Street, then enter Pier 41 on your right. Visit whichever art and design tenants pique your interest. Down the pier on the south side is Red Hook Winery and its lively tasting room.

Go back to the inland end of the pier and onto the path between the water and the picket-fence-enclosed Liberty Garden (source of produce for the Liberty Warehouse). You can walk on a concrete path or the boardwalk at the water's edge; either will bring you to a grassy area with boulders and benches—and another great view of the Statue of Liberty. Then proceed to the Lehigh Valley railroad barge at the next pier, home of the ❻ Waterfront Museum, full of nautical artifacts. Special maritime-themed exhibits, as well as concerts and theatrical productions, are also held onboard. From the end of this pier, look to your right at Pier 41 and to your left at the Beard Street Warehouse (and the Verrazano-Narrows Bridge). They're the only brick-warehouse piers remaining from Brooklyn's shipping heyday, when the waterfront all the way north to the Queens border was lined with such wharves.

From the Waterfront Museum, cross the parking lot to Conover Street and make a left. At Reed Street, you can see ahead to a generic BAR sign hanging from a building on your right. That is Sunny's, the sole surviving longshoremen's bar on a strip that once had some 40 such establishments. The big coffeepots where workers used to fill up for their morning jolt are still kept behind the bar.

Turn right on Reed, passing the private home at #26 covered driveway-to-roof with buoys, mounted fish, and other nautical bric-a-brac. Two of Red Hook's destination restaurants fill out the block: Brooklyn Crab and Hometown Bar-B-Que. Upon reaching Van Brunt Street, you're facing the Beard Street Warehouse. If you go to the right, you can read about its history on a sign outside #499, which is the section actually on the pier. Old photos and artifacts are on display in its lobby.

Look for the Beard & Robinson nameplate below the top right window of #481, the warehouse opposite Fairway. Beneath it, at Door 7, the Brooklyn Waterfront Artists Coalition (BWAC) has an exhibition space. Heading back toward Reed Street, you can stop in any open artist studios or design showrooms.

Past Reed Street, Ample Hills Creamery has a new production facility at 421 Van Brunt, which should be open for tours as of spring 2018. Ample Hills plans to have one of its signature churning bikes installed then too, so you can assist in making the ice cream. Or just eat it.

Turn right at Van Dyke Street. At the end of the block on your left is an 1859 structure described as "basilica-like" in its landmark designation—which was a first for Red Hook. This storehouse for the Brooklyn Clay Retort and Fire Brick Works, a company that both manufactured bricks *and* was owned by a man named Brick, is made of stones nearly 2 feet thick.

Turn left at Dwight Street. The six-point star above a door on your left marks the home of Sixpoint Brewery, here since 2004. About 10 more breweries have opened in the borough since then—still, not quite the 50 or so that were based in Brooklyn at the turn of the century.

Turn right on Coffey.

Make a left on Otsego Street and a quick right on Bay Street for the ❼ **Van Brunt Stillhouse,** producer of whiskeys, bourbon, rum, and the Korean spirit *soju*. A cocktail bar adjoins its distillery.

Retracing your steps from the distillery, make a left from Bay Street onto Otsego Street. After crossing Sigourney Street, you're walking beside the Red Hook Community Farm—it took the place of a rundown playground in the early 2000s. Young people who work at the farm and its composting operation receive job training and education in sustainable agriculture and food service.

Turn right at Beard Street.

Go left at the traffic light and IKEA banners, and follow the sidewalk past the parking lot and into ❽ **Erie Basin Park,** created by IKEA in exchange for the rezoning that allowed it to build its store. In addition to landscaping and assorted seating, the park features displays of cranes, bollards, ropes, and other shipping-related relics—many of them salvaged from the Todd Shipyard, which was shut down after 150 years in business to clear the way for IKEA.

Cap off your visit to this harbor-side community with a ferry ride (on which you'll get a great alternative view of where you've just been). The water-taxi dock is right here in Erie Basin Park. If you want to travel by land, the bus stop is in front of IKEA on Beard Street.

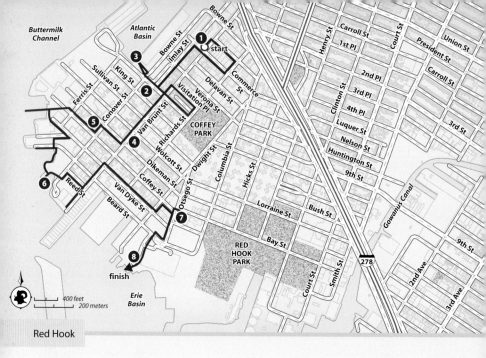

Points of Interest

1 Raaka Virgin Chocolate 64 Seabring St.; 855-255-3354, raakachocolate.com

2 Pioneer Works 159 Pioneer St.; 718-596-3001, pioneerworks.org

3 PortSide NewYork/*Mary A. Whalen* Bowne Street and Pioneer Street; 917-414-0565, portsidenewyork.org

4 Kentler International Drawing Space 353 Van Brunt St.; 718-875-2098, kentlergallery.org

5 Cacao Prieto and Widow Jane Distillery 218 Conover St.; 347-225-0130, cacaoprieto.com and widowjane.com

6 Waterfront Museum 290 Conover St.; 718-624-4719, waterfrontmuseum.org

7 Van Brunt Stillhouse 6 Bay St.; 718-852-6405, vanbruntstillhouse.com

8 Erie Basin Park 1 Beard St.

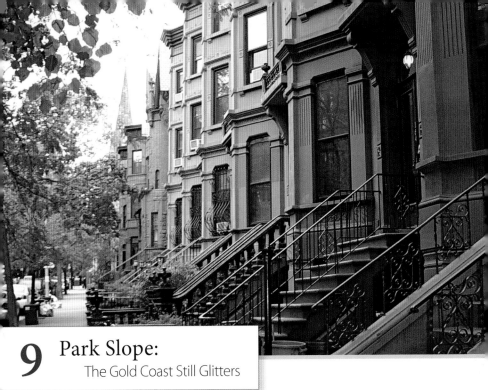

9 Park Slope:
The Gold Coast Still Glitters

Above: Memorial Presbyterian's spire caps a brownstone block of St. John's Place

BOUNDARIES: Sterling Pl., Prospect Park W., 4th St., 6th Ave.
DISTANCE: 2.6 miles
SUBWAY: 2 or 3 to Grand Army Plaza (Plaza St. W. exit)

Park Slope was ahead of the curve when it came to gentrification. It was rediscovered during the brownstone revival of the late 1960s, so it's been a coveted address for some time. The millionaires who transformed it into Brooklyn's "Gold Coast" after Prospect Park and the Brooklyn Bridge opened in the late 1800s left behind a dazzling array of mansions and townhouses in Romanesque, Queen Anne, Italianate, and Renaissance Revival styles. That classic Brooklyn image of brownstone rowhouses with stoops is found on street after street of Park Slope. Brooklyn also gained its reputation as the "city of churches" from neighborhoods like this. The latter-day citizenry has elicited resentment and mocking for their overindulgent parenting, overpriced lifestyles, and seeming homogeneity, but others dismiss such negativity merely as real estate envy. Park Slope, after all, is one of America's Victorian treasures, with a vibrant commercial component and proximity to the park, botanic garden, and Brooklyn Museum.

Walk Description

Walk one block on Plaza Street West in the same direction that cars travel. On your right at Lincoln Place, you have your first encounter with the grande dame of Park Slope, the ❶ **Montauk Club.** Its fairy tale–ish two-story curved bay (with balcony on top) would alone impress, but turn right on Lincoln to see the rest of this amazing Victorian Gothic Venetian palazzo, opened in 1891. Near the top, a terra cotta frieze illustrating Montauk Indian history wraps around to the 8th Avenue facade—follow it to see an additional frieze on the front of the building that depicts the club's founders laying the cornerstone. This was one of the first men's clubs to let wives in, and that second front door, to the left, was the women's entrance; it led directly to stairs up to the dining room, so ladies could bypass the lobby. Note the Native American heads peering down at the main entrance. There is still a club inside, but membership is not exclusionary. On the other side of 8th Avenue, #22 has what are known as City Hall lamps, indicating a mayor has lived there. The mayor was William Jay Gaynor, who was shot in an assassination attempt not long after taking office in 1910 and died of his injuries . . . three years later!

Make a left on St. John's Place. Lots of brownstone on this long block; toward the end on your left, #212 was Gaynor's home before he moved around the corner (and was elected mayor). Over on your right, the picturesque elements of Grace United Methodist include flying buttresses. This church stands diagonally across 7th Avenue from Memorial Presbyterian—built in the same style, Victorian Gothic, around the same time, 1882, but looking completely different. Memorial Presbyterian has stained-glass windows by Tiffany.

After crossing 7th Avenue, you pass yet another church, quaint St. John's Episcopal. Both its chapel and rectory date to 1870, and they're enhanced by a garden. Across the street, note the red gable embossed with a caduceus, the intertwining-snakes symbol of the medical profession. The first owner of this house, in 1888, was a doctor.

Turn right on 6th Avenue. ❷ **St. Augustine,** on the left at Sterling Place, is considered the masterpiece of the Parfitt Brothers, who designed a number of illustrious Brooklyn churches, including Grace United. Towers, spires, and lancet windows abound in this phenomenal church, which is crowned with a copper statue of the angel Gabriel blowing his trumpet.

With the church to your left, head up Sterling Place. Look up at the apartment house at #126—bricks above the top windows are a different color from those below. That's because this building had to be repaired after a United Airlines jetliner crashed into it on December 16, 1960. The pilot was trying to make an emergency landing in Prospect Park after colliding midair in fog with a TWA plane, which then crashed on Staten Island. Everybody aboard both flights died, and six people on the street in Park Slope were killed, including two men selling Christmas trees on the sidewalk—the death toll of 134 made it the world's worst commercial aviation disaster to date. (An 11-year-old boy was the only victim not pronounced dead at the scene; he died the next day at Methodist Hospital on 6th Street, where a memorial plaque in the chapel is affixed with his pocket change.) A church on the northwest corner of Sterling and 7th Avenue (to your left) was destroyed in the plane crash, but miraculously, the mansion catercorner from it was spared serious damage. For a pick-me-up after this grim story, turn your attention to that mansion, with a delightful oriel protruding from the corner. Its entrance is on Sterling, but it was built as a set with the three houses next to it on 7th Avenue.

Go to your right on 7th. The corner mansion on the right as you reach Lincoln Place now belongs to the ❸ **Brooklyn Conservatory of Music** (founded in 1897), which sponsors a community chorale and a symphony orchestra in addition to holding classes and private lessons.

Turn right on Lincoln. The formidable Romanesque mansion at #153 was converted to a condominium after being sold in 2007, but somehow it had been left alone for the previous 40-odd years—while the neighborhood filled with wealth and children—even though everyone knew a hot-sheet hotel was operating inside. One tryst ended in murder in 1999, when a woman was hanged from the shower rod by her lover. The 1887 home's original owner was Frank L. Babbott, art collector, proprietor of a fiber mill, and son-in-law of oilman Charles Pratt.

Make a left on 6th, then a left on Union Street. About halfway down on your right is the Park Slope Food Coop, established in 1973, well before terms like *organic* and *macrobiotic* became part of everyone's dietary lexicon. More than a few of its internecine controversies—over issues ranging from sourcing of merchandise to members' attempts to evade the monthly work requirement—have gone public. Next door is the station house of Squad 1, an elite rescue unit of the FDNY that lost 12 men on 9/11. The memorial outside the firehouse, based on the iconic photograph from Ground Zero, was crafted from spruce trees by a sculptor and volunteer fireman in Portland, Oregon.

Make a right on 7th Avenue. At Carroll Street, the ❹ **Old First Reformed Church** serves a congregation established in the 17th century. It's had four previous homes around Brooklyn.

Turn left on Carroll, and a symmetrical quartet of homes greets you past the bank on the right, its two middle homes united by a bracketed ledge above their doors and first-floor windows.

Turn right onto Polhemus Place. The homes in the longer row on your left have charming floral ornamentation around their doors and lower windows.

Go left onto Garfield Place. At 8th Avenue, cross over to the domed Neoclassical synagogue of **❺ Congregation Beth Elohim** on the left. Then turn to the more modern building opposite Garfield Place—the congregation's temple house, where Moses stands atop the corner with the Ten Commandments.

Walk south on 8th Avenue. Past the brownstones on your right, spend a few moments examining the triangular gables of two limestone houses—see the small busts between their windows? The corner house lost a similar gable when a floor was added. A conical roof caps the corner at the end of the next block, and another peak rises across 2nd Street at the Byzantine Melkite Church of the Virgin Mary, where Catholics of Arab descent have worshipped since 1952. The house next to it is atypical for the neighborhood—neither a mansion nor a brownstone townhouse, it looks like it was designed for a country or suburban setting. It was built in 1913 by the Neergaard family, who founded a Park Slope pharmacy in 1888 that's still in business.

Turn left on 4th Street. Upon reaching Prospect Park West, you'll be facing **❻ Litchfield Villa**, which stands inside Prospect Park. It was built in 1857—on a hill, to give it a view of the harbor—as the home of Edwin Litchfield, a man who made his fortune on land speculation but ironically ran into a quandary over his own property. He was forced to sell the villa to the city of Brooklyn when the park was created, then rent it back. Go down the drive on the right to the colonnade between the mansion and its newer annex. The columns have corncob capitals to honor the country's agrarian past (they're also found on columns in the United States Capitol). The parks department has offices inside the house, and you should be able to enter during business hours.

Walk on Prospect Park West with the park on your right. Its 3rd Street entrance is guarded by two identical panthers . . . identical except for one feature—can you spot it? (See page 58.) Then turn to the residential side of Prospect Park West. 2nd Street is flanked by two designs of William Tubby, a favorite architect of Brooklyn's smart set at the turn of the century. William Childs, founder of the Bon Ami scouring powder brand, hired Tubby in 1910 for the house at #61 that Childs gave his daughter as a wedding present. Ten years earlier, Tubby had designed Childs's own mansion at #53.

The gigantic 1889 house next door (now a private school) was designed by another great Gilded Age architect, Montrose Morris. It looks symmetrical at first glance, but the tower on the left is smaller and rounded compared to the polygonal right tower, and the doors are not centered but skewed to the left (the arch on the right is a window).

Feel free to divert your eyes to the Grand Army Plaza arch, ahead down Prospect Park West. The man who commissioned the chariot statue atop the arch lived in the brownstone and brick house at #32, just north of Garfield Place. His name was Frank Squier, and he was appointed parks commissioner of Brooklyn in 1895.

Dutch Treats

While there's no denying the allure of Park Slope and other brownstone neighborhoods' 19th-century homes, Brooklyn's housing stock goes back another 200-plus years. The borough's oldest residence, now operating as the **Wyckoff House Museum** (5816 Clarendon Road; 718-629-5400, wyckoffmuseum.org), was built around 1652 by Pieter Claesen Wyckoff. Situated at Canarsie's border with East Flatbush, where Ralph and Ditmas Avenues intersect, the Wyckoff property is beautifully preserved and presents a vivid history lesson, with period objects and furnishings in the rooms and a working farm on premises. Two of Brooklyn's other extant colonial-era farmhouses are not museums themselves, but are *in* the Brooklyn Museum. Both the circa-1676 Jan Martense Schenck House and the Nicholas Schenck House from the early 1770s were dismantled, then reassembled in their entirety as exhibitions in the museum's decorative arts galleries.

Turn left on Montgomery Place, described by one architectural historian as a "great urban ensemble." Its initial development in 1887–88 comprised #11, 17, and 19 on your right and #14–16 facing them. They launched the career of their 24-year-old architect, Charles P. H. Gilbert, who's responsible for nearly half the houses on this block (including #36–60). Take your time observing ornamental detail on all these homes, or just wallowing in the picture-perfect milieu.

Turn right on 8th Avenue for a queue of spectacular mansions and finely appointed apartment buildings. Some need to be seen from the side street as well as the avenue, such as the reddish-brown behemoth on your right at Carroll Street, which could be called the House That Chiclets Built. Thomas Adams Jr. didn't afford this home on his brand of gum alone; he also invented a coin-operated machine for its convenient, widespread sale. This double house, now subdivided into apartments, has stained-glass panes above every window and is supposedly haunted by servants who died in its elevator after it malfunctioned.

A couple of doors down, #105 is one of the newer kids on the block, built around 1912. The elegant apartment building next to it was also built as a single-family home, in 1909, for a brewery executive. Past President Street, watch on the left for the knights in armor aside #78's bay window. On your left across Union Street, the corner house's cylindrical tower produces an almost comic effect. Both this manse and the one at the other end of the block, at Berkeley, quirkily mesh materials, architectural styles, and geometric forms.

Make a right on Berkeley Place, then go left on Plaza Street West for two blocks to the subway station where you began.

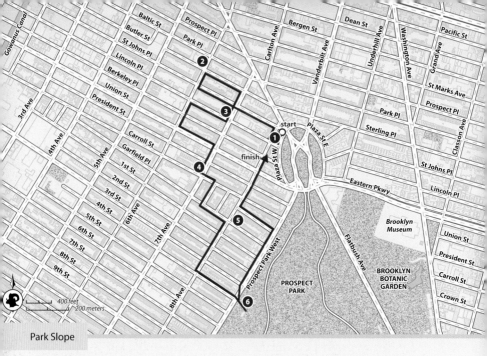

Points of Interest

1. **Montauk Club** 25 8th Ave.; 718-638-0800, montaukclub.com
2. **St. Augustine** 116 6th Ave.; 718-783-3132, staugustineparkslope.org
3. **Brooklyn Conservatory of Music** 58 7th Ave.; 718-622-3300, bkcm.org
4. **Old First Reformed Church** 729 Carroll St.; 718-638-8300, oldfirstbrooklyn.org
5. **Congregation Beth Elohim** 274 Garfield Place; 718-768-3814, congregationbethelohim.org
6. **Litchfield Villa** Prospect Park West and 5th Street; 718-965-8900

ANSWER: What's different about the panthers? Their ears.

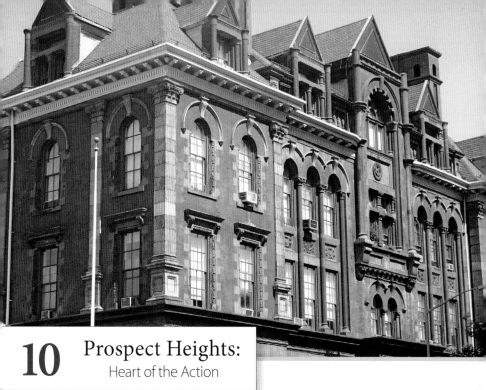

10 Prospect Heights:
Heart of the Action

Above: The former P.S. 9 annex

BOUNDARIES: Putnam Ave., Franklin Ave., Eastern Pkwy., Flatbush Ave.
DISTANCE: 3.8 miles
SUBWAY: B or Q to 7th Ave. (Flatbush Ave. exit)

Prospect Heights may be the richest neighborhood in Brooklyn. Not in income, but in institutions. It's home to three of the borough's most beloved: the Brooklyn Museum, Brooklyn Public Library, and Brooklyn Botanic Garden. The area around Eastern Parkway where they're located is still sometimes referred to as Institute Park, after the museum's original name, the Brooklyn Institute of Arts and Sciences. Prospect Heights has both a Victorian historic district and ultra-modern, innovative housing: modular, or prefab, high-rises in the new Pacific Park development that feature luxury amenities in subsidized "affordable" buildings. This route begins with residential Prospect Heights, then dips into bordering neighborhoods as it wends toward the cultural heart of Brooklyn around the museum.

Walk Description

Do a 180 at the top of the subway stairs so you're walking with the Flatbush Avenue roadbed to your left. Cross Sterling Place and enjoy the view of the building diagonally across the intersection: an 1885 brownstone, half on Flatbush, half on Sterling, its central tower aligned precisely with the corner. A widow's walk caps the tower's pyramidal slate roof, and even it is crowned with finials. Lower down on the tower, see the wrought-iron balcony and original wood door.

Now cross Flatbush and walk on Sterling. At the end of the block, P.S. 340 (originally P.S. 9) is a little red schoolhouse from 1868. Too little, it turned out. Following the opening of Prospect Park and the Brooklyn Bridge, the neighborhood's population had grown so much that an annex had to be built. Cross Vanderbilt Avenue to see that rather grand "annex," completed in 1895. It's the alma mater of *Appalachian Spring* composer Aaron Copland but has been residential since the '80s.

Turn back and make a right on Vanderbilt Avenue, heading north.

Turn left on Prospect Place. The homes around here are not only lovely but historic—among the earliest rowhouses in the neighborhood. The houses at #210 and #198 through 190 are from the late 1860s.

Turn right on Carlton Avenue, where the first couple of houses on both sides are pre-1870. Cross St. Mark's Avenue for the residences thought to be the oldest in the neighborhood: the pair of three-story houses on your left standing alone between yards. They were erected between 1850 and 1855, and the iron fence around them is believed to be original.

At the next corner on your right, what appears to be a great Romanesque mansion is actually three separate houses, built as an ensemble in 1893. To your left, the two houses flanking Bergen look similar but were built at different times by different architects. In fact, #560 and #558—built together in 1882—are suspected of copying the houses next to them. If it's true, then the adage "steal from the best" kicked in, as #556–550 are the work of the Parfitt Brothers, whose illustrious output includes Grace United and St. Augustine churches nearby in Park Slope. On the left corner at Dean Street is a fabulously frilly turn-of-the-century house. Look atop the window above the door: amid the floral carving is a shield with an *R*—for Reilly, the first family to live here.

Make a left on Dean Street. Past some brownstones on your right, the condominium with a color-blocked entry is called Newswalk—this building was a *Daily News* printing plant from 1927 to 1997. We'll take the pattern within the iron fence as another homage, as it seems inspired by printers' boxes (that held typesetting keys). Farther down, the Temple of Restoration worships in a building erected in 1893 as a Swedish Baptist Church, a reminder of Brooklyn's once robust Scandinavian population.

Go into the playground across the street and follow the path straight through to Bergen Street. Go to your right on Bergen. Take in the massive Peter F. Reilly's Warehouse & Vaults building on the right. Remember the *R* house on Carlton Avenue? He's the Reilly who owned it.

Turn right on 6th Avenue, coming around to the front of the ❶ **NYPD's 78th Precinct**— which you may recognize as the "99th Precinct" on *Brooklyn Nine-Nine*. Hollywood likes this station house: it also starred on the Debra Messing series *The Mysteries of Laura* and the 1990s cop drama *Brooklyn South*.

Savor this last bit of old Prospect Heights before you cross Dean Street and the new Prospect Heights soars before you. On the left corner across Dean rises a 23-story "affordable" building that's part of the Pacific Park megadevelopment. The building with red that you see behind it farther down Dean is another Pacific Park residence and also happens to be the world's tallest modular building—made off-site and assembled in sections, akin to "a giant Lego set," per one local blog. Pacific Park is the residential component of what was long referred to as the "Atlantic Yards project." It started with the construction of Barclays Center, the back of which you see here on 6th Avenue.

Turn right on Pacific. Down on your left is the Vanderbilt Yard, as the MTA calls it, which was rebranded the Atlantic Yards by the developer who bought up more than 20 acres surrounding it in 2005–06. He wanted to build an arena so he could move the New Jersey Nets, whom he'd also recently purchased, to Brooklyn. It ballooned into a $5 billion, eminent-domain-invoking plan for 16 additional buildings, including a Frank Gehry–designed skyscraper. Years of demonstrations and lawsuits—even an off-Broadway play critical of it—tainted the name Atlantic Yards, and by the time the scaled-down project (no more Gehry, among other things) broke ground on its residential buildings, it had gotten a new name, Pacific Park.

Continue past the back of the Newswalk building and cross Carlton Avenue. To your right is another Pacific Park building. Rents in both this one and the building at Dean and 6th are below market rate, and the 300 apartments in each are all distributed based on a lottery that people could enter if they had an eligible income: between $20,126 and . . . $173,415! Whereas most affordable housing is just for lower-income residents, these also have an allotment for "moderate" and "middle-income." This block is all Pacific Park property. At press time, six residential buildings had been announced in total—four rental, two condominium. More are expected, and so are more twists and turns in this saga. Remember, this all sprang from the developer's acquisition of the Nets. Well, they do play in Brooklyn now, but he doesn't own them anymore.

Upon crossing Vanderbilt, you leave the "new" Prospect Heights behind and see before you the ❷ **Co-Cathedral of St. Joseph.** In one of his last acts as pope, Benedict XVI elevated St. Joseph to co- status with St. James on Jay Street (which was already designated a cathedral) in February

2013, after the diocese decided that it is more centrally located to the population than the smaller St. James. Go inside if you can, or just gaze at the expressive cherubim on the exterior.

Make a left at Underhill Avenue, then head through Lowry Triangle on your right, pausing at the bust to read about its namesake minister. The tip of the triangle is a good vantage point for the flamboyant building across Atlantic Avenue with multiple verdigris towers. This was Cathedral College, a seminary *and* seminary prep school for young men considering the priesthood. Its two most famous alumni never made it to ordination: chef Rocco DiSpirito and NFL coach Vince Lombardi. The school moved to Queens in the 1980s, and the building became a condominium not long after.

Cross Atlantic Avenue and go to the right in front of the Cathedral building. Look for the gargoyles flying out from it.

Turn left on St. James Place, entering Clinton Hill as you move north of Atlantic.

Make a right on Lefferts Place. This block of brownstones and brickfronts concludes with a Second Empire–style mini-mansion on your right that has a quaint "bump-out" on the Grand Avenue side. Continue across Grand to the first freestanding house on your right, #70. It's pretty much the only freestanding house like this in the area, a landmarked villa from 1854. For about 50 years beginning in 1939, this was a residence for followers of Father Divine and local base for his International Peace Mission.

Go back to Grand Avenue and turn right, walking alongside an ornate church busy with windows and wings in a multitude of shapes. Seek out the wonderful terra cotta carving at the tops of the rectangular towers and elsewhere on this 1880s edifice.

Make a right on Putnam Avenue. On your left after Irving Place, a fraternal organization has its headquarters in the vertiginous landmark structure built for the ❸ **Lincoln Club,** an organization of Republicans, in 1889. The club's initials interlock on the gable beside the bullet-shaped half-tower of this Renaissance–Romanesque mélange.

Turn right on Classon Avenue, then left onto Lefferts Place, a block with an interesting assortment of homes, including a contiguous sextet with picturesque oriel windows on the right.

Make a right on Franklin Avenue. By this point you are within the bounds of Bedford-Stuyvesant—at least according to some people (neighborhood borders are debatable). Cross Atlantic Avenue, and now it's Crown Heights.

Make a right at Bergen Street. Though the building on your right bears the name of its later commercial tenant, Heinz, it was built for the Nassau Brewery, which operated from 1849 to 1914 and went through a succession of earlier names, including Budwiser—which sparked a lawsuit from Anheuser-Busch. The street's beer heritage stays alive on the other side of the train trestle, where the combination food hall and beer garden ❹ **Berg'n** opened in a former garage in 2014.

Make a left on Classon Avenue and head to Eastern Parkway. Frederick Law Olmsted and Calvert Vaux created Eastern Parkway and its pedestrian mall as part of their Prospect Park design and of a grander plan to link NYC parks with landscaped boulevards and green spaces. That vision was unfulfilled, but their felicitous concept for this, the world's first six-lane parkway, earned it recognition by the National Register of Historic Places and the city landmarks commission.

Cross Eastern Parkway and go right into Dr. Ronald McNair Park. Proceed to the three-sided obelisk that displays bronze images of the Challenger astronaut and his accomplishments, and inscriptions of his thoughts on the universe.

Head back to Eastern Parkway via the park's other path, which puts you at Washington Avenue. Cross Washington, and now you're definitely back in Prospect Heights. But more importantly, you've reached the ❺ **Brooklyn Museum**! At the foot of the bleachers here, you'll want to watch the dancing waters in the fountain. The building itself is a Beaux Arts stunner from 1893, its entrance flanked by allegorical female sculptures by Daniel Chester French, of Lincoln Memorial fame. They represent Manhattan and (with the boy) Brooklyn. The Brooklyn Museum's world-class holdings span all eras and cultures. Highlights include the Egyptian antiquities (some say the best collection outside Cairo); decorative objects and period rooms; the American galleries; art of the Islamic world; and the Elizabeth A. Sackler Center for Feminist Art, with Judy Chicago's *The Dinner Party* as its centerpiece. The museum also has more than 20 Rodin sculptures, Impressionist paintings, and a sculpture garden full of architectural salvage. And even with its international reach, the museum never loses sight of the local community, frequently staging exhibitions showcasing New York artists or themes.

There's a subway station on the west side of the museum plaza. Or add on this short extension (quarter of a mile):

Proceed west along the same side of Eastern Parkway. You'll pass an entrance to the Brooklyn Botanic Garden (see page 76). Just after that, follow the path into Mount Prospect Park. This is the second-highest point in Brooklyn and was used as a lookout by the Continental Army during the Revolutionary War. It was turned into a park after Olmsted and Vaux nixed its inclusion in Prospect Park because they didn't want a section of Flatbush Avenue running through it. Still, Prospect Park took its name from Mount Prospect. Walk on the path to the next exit (down steps) to Eastern Parkway. To your left is the central branch of the ❻ **Brooklyn Public Library.** This concludes the extension, though you could continue to Grand Army Plaza or Prospect Park (see Walk 11) or even Park Slope (Walk 9).

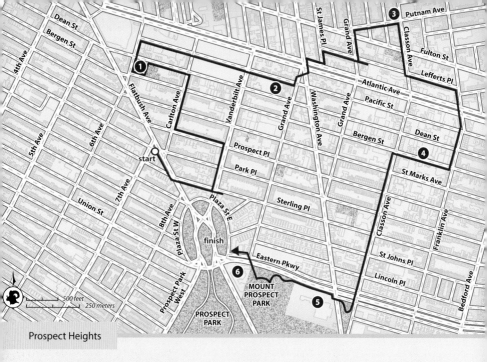

Points of Interest

1. **NYPD 78th Precinct** 65 6th Ave., 718-636-6411, nyc.gov/html/nypd/html/precincts/precinct_078.shtml

2. **Co-Cathedral of St. Joseph** 856 Pacific St.; 718-638-1071, stjosephs-brooklyn.org

3. **Lincoln Club** 65 Putnam Ave.; 718-789-2105

4. **Berg'n** 899 Bergen St.; bergn.com

5. **Brooklyn Museum** 200 Eastern Parkway; 718-638-5000, brooklynmuseum.org

6. **Brooklyn Public Library** 10 Grand Army Plaza; 718-230-2100, bklynlibrary.org

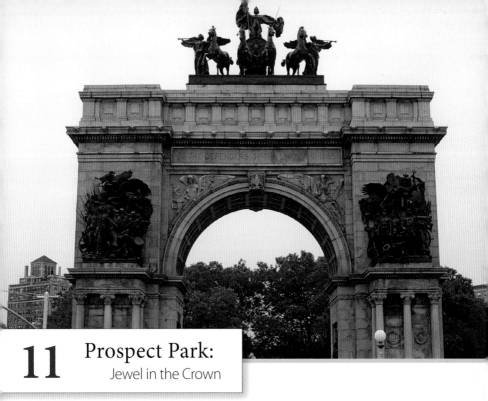

11 Prospect Park:
Jewel in the Crown

BOUNDARIES: Plaza St. E., East Dr., lake, Prospect Park W.
DISTANCE: Approx. 4.5 miles
SUBWAY: 2 or 3 to Grand Army Plaza (Plaza St. E. and Vanderbilt Ave. exit)

Frederick Law Olmsted and Calvert Vaux, pioneers of landscape architecture and the urban parks movement in the United States, are most famous for Central Park but were prouder of Prospect Park. When they'd designed Central Park a decade earlier, they were frustrated by certain requirements, such as the rectangular shape and the flattening of rolling land. Freed of such constraints for Prospect Park, Olmsted and Vaux created a park they considered more naturalistic. Before construction commenced in the 1860s, Brooklynites had only Green-Wood Cemetery and 30-acre Washington (now Fort Greene) Park for a bucolic escape. By the time Prospect Park was completed in 1873, they would find within its 526 acres a natural forest, meadows, small hills, and a series of waterways coursing through the eastern half and emptying into a lake. The park also contains some notable statuary and architecture, as well as historic sites and recreational attractions.

Walk Description

The angel-themed artwork in the subway station is an homage to the angels atop the ❶ **Grand Army Plaza** arch, which you'll soon see. Exit the subway at Plaza Street East and Vanderbilt Avenue, using the stairs on the right. At street level, walk straight ahead. With the bust of Alexander J. C. Skene (a Union Army surgeon and later a pioneering gynecologist) on your left, cross the street. Then go to your right, crossing two sections of the traffic circle until you come face-to-face with John F. Kennedy. This bust is, surprisingly, the rare monument to JFK in this Democratic city with a sizable Irish-Catholic population. Proceed to Bailey Fountain, where a man and woman representing Wisdom and Felicity stand in the center. At their pedestal, Tritons blow conch shells, and facing the arch is Neptune, god of the sea. Look for the chubby child and his horn of plenty at the man's right knee.

As you head to the triumphal arch, look to your left and right at the statues ringing the traffic circle. That's General Slocum on horseback; he's remembered more as the namesake of an ill-fated steamboat—the 1904 fire aboard it killed 1,021 people, a death toll second only to 9/11 among NYC disasters—than for his service in the Civil War (and later Congress). Over on your right, the statue of the standing man is Gouverneur Kemble Warren, another Civil War general; he's remembered more as the brother of Emily Roebling, who shepherded construction of the Brooklyn Bridge after her husband, chief engineer Washington Roebling, was incapacitated by illness.

Proceed through the Soldiers' and Sailors' Memorial Arch, then turn around to look at it. You'll see the Union Army depicted in the sculptural grouping on the left, the Navy on the right. Take a few minutes to study these stirring tributes. Note the fallen: a soldier lying prone before the angel in the Army tableau, a sailor slumped on the left side of the Navy group. Frederick MacMonnies, the sculptor, used himself as the model for the Army officer brandishing a sword at front. He also included a black man in the Navy scene (crouching next to the cannon), making this one of the few Civil War monuments to portray an African American. The arch is topped by a sculpture of a quadriga, a four-horse chariot, ridden by Columbia (representing the United States) and two angels of victory.

With your back to the arch, you have a fine view to your left of the 40-foot-high doors of the main branch of the Brooklyn Public Library, which feature bronze sculptings of literary characters and authors. The two women in the top row are Hester Prynne (left) and *Little Women*'s Meg March. Tom Sawyer's at the bottom left, Rip Van Winkle two panels above him. The animals include Moby Dick, Edgar Allan Poe's raven, and a howling White Fang from the Jack London novel. Walt

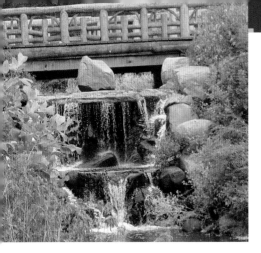

Binnen Bridge and Binnen Falls get their name from the Dutch word for "within"

Whitman is depicted above Wynken, Blynken, and Nod in their wooden-shoe boat. You can even see from this vantage point that the building is shaped like an open book.

Note: *Walking directions within the park refer to trails, paths, and drives. Drives are blacktop roads with separate lanes for pedestrians, bicycles, and vehicles. Paths are also paved, but they're meant for foot traffic only. Trails are unpaved and usually in the woods.*

Cross over to the main entrance of Prospect Park, heralded by four eagle-topped columns. Follow the path between the two columns on the left, tipping your hat to the "Father of Prospect Park," James Stranahan, depicted in a statue by Frederick MacMonnies. Stranahan not only spearheaded creation of the park, but was also involved in other major civic projects of the time, including the building of the Brooklyn Bridge.

Stay on the path as it takes you under Endale Arch. This is Brooklyn's oldest bridge, still standing from when the park was created in 1867. Its name was compressed from "enter dale," which is what you do as you come out the other side at the edge of Long Meadow. This was all part of Olmsted and Vaux's vision of the park as a place where people are distanced from urban sights and sounds.

Take the path to your right. The trees on your right comprise the 9/11 Grove, a "living memorial."

When you reach Meadowport Arch, you can do an in-one, out-the-other, as Olmsted designed it with a double opening onto Long Meadow.

Walk on the grass to the other side of Long Meadow and make a right. Head up the concrete staircase on your left, then turn right on East Drive. On your left, after passing a lawn, watch for a boulder beside a tree identifying the Continental Army's line of defense during the Battle of Long Island, aka the Battle of Brooklyn. Just after it, a boulder to your right bears a plaque about Battle Pass. Continuing on East Drive, just before the traffic light you'll find on your left an eagle monument where an oak tree was cut down and thrown in the way of advancing British troops.

Take the East Drive sidewalk heading away from Dongan Oak. Stay on that path till you behold the carousel, built in 1912 and moved into the park from—where else?—Coney Island. The old white farmhouse here in the Children's Corner, ❷ **Lefferts Historic House,** was also relocated into the park; it was constructed in the 1780s on Flatbush Avenue, about half a mile from here, and now serves as a museum of 1820s farm life. The path in front leads to the ❸ **Prospect Park Zoo.** On the side of the carousel away from the Lefferts House, take the center path (with arrows pointing toward the Boathouse and other places). Follow it down and through Eastwood Arch. With the Boathouse to your left, go right onto Binnen Bridge.

Across the bridge, note the Music Pagoda on your right—a circa-1970 reconstruction of an 1880s structure once famous for its brass-band concerts. But go down the path on your left to the viewing platform for the Boathouse and Binnen Falls. A lean-to sufficed as the boathouse in the park's early years; this gorgeous replacement, modeled on the Sansoviniana library in St. Mark's square in Venice, was built in 1905. From there, walk alongside the water and then up the path leading onto Lullwater Bridge.

As you step off Lullwater Bridge on its other end, note the arbor across the water to your right. Several such "rustic shelters" were erected in the park, reintroducing a feature from the Olmsted–Vaux plan. The shelters were made with no nails, only pegs and dowels holding the logs together. Off the bridge, take the first path on your left to the Boathouse so you can see its terra cotta detail close-up, enjoy a view of the Lullwater from the terrace, and go inside if the Boathouse is open. The first urban ❹ **Audubon Center** in the country was established here; Prospect Park was an apt choice, as it's home to some 260 species of birds.

Leave the Boathouse on the side where you entered, but follow the path to your left. Not far along on your left is the squat and gnarly Camperdown Elm, planted in 1872 and now protected by a fence. There are fewer than 10 such trees in the world—Mr. Camperdown made just a handful of cuttings of his elm in Scotland that, due to a mutation, grew low and parallel to the ground instead of upright. Like the Boathouse, this tree was once slated for removal; preservation efforts for both were led by poet and Brooklyn resident Marianne Moore, who penned an ode to the elm.

Head past the elm and through Cleft Ridge Arch. Go right and walk to the Oriental Pavilion ahead on your left. Originally built in 1874 for concert audiences, it was eventually converted to a snack bar—which went up in flames in 1974. Only the cast-iron pillars survived the fire and are part of this reconstruction. Don't miss the stained-glass skylight at the center.

From the pavilion, head down the steps into the Concert Grove and wander amid its busts of Mozart, Beethoven, and other composers. Leave the Concert Grove on the side where you see buildings outside the park (you will eventually loop around to the sights on the other side). Down the stairs and across the drive, see a bust of Washington Irving, native New Yorker and author of "The Legend of Sleepy Hollow." Facing Irving, make a right and proceed to Imagination Playground, where another local writer is honored: Ezra Jack Keats, the award-winning children's book author who was born and raised in Brooklyn. Peter and his dog Willie, two of Keats's recurring characters, are represented, along with two of the books in which they appear, *A Snowy Day* and *Peter's Chair*.

Come out of the playground and go left on the sidewalk. When you reach the Drummer's Grove (created after a West Indian drumming circle had been meeting at the spot for years) on your left, cross East Drive and proceed, via grass or path, to the lake. Walk with the lake on your left and the ❺ **LeFrak Center at Lakeside** on your right. It has connected indoor and outdoor skating rinks, the latter of which transforms into a "splash pad" in the summer. Continuing along, watch for the World War I memorial on your left. Loss rather than heroism sets the mood, accentuated by the veiled angel of death at the center. Brooklyn's casualties are listed on honor roll tablets crafted by Daniel Chester French, sculptor of the Lincoln Memorial.

Speaking of President Lincoln . . . you'll soon meet up with him if you keep walking beside the lake. This statue of the president holding the Emancipation Proclamation was created for Grand Army Plaza in 1868 and moved into the park in 1895.

This spot gives you a feel for what park planners intended for the Concert Grove. People used to sit in the Oriental Pavilion or on the grass while the musicians occupied a stage on an island in the lake. A new "music island" was created in the development of the LeFrak Center at Lakeside (which opened in 2013), but it's strictly a wildlife habitat. There haven't been regular performances here since the 1890s, mainly due to poor acoustics.

Turn away from Lincoln and walk to your right, continuing on the path beside the lake. It leads right onto a path into the woods. Follow it uphill, and then cross Terrace Bridge on your left. Beneath you, the Lullwater flows into the lake.

Once across the bridge, scale Lookout Hill—where you see the column with a sphere on top. This monument honors the Maryland 400, a volunteer regiment who engaged British soldiers in a skirmish at the nearby Old Stone House (featured in Walk 7).

Go back down the hill and to your right on Wellhouse Drive. The structure that gave this road its name will soon appear on your right. This brick hut, designed by Calvert Vaux in 1869, held the pumps that fed the lake from a well 70 feet underground. It became obsolete when the park hooked up to the city's water supply, and was recently refurbished as a restroom with the first composting toilets in an NYC park.

Not far past the Wellhouse are picnic tables; walk up the hilly lawn behind them, and at the top go right on the path (*not* on the drive that bicyclists use). A short way in, instead of using steps to the right, go left onto the woodsy trail. It too ascends; take it to where it reaches a black-top drive, and then turn right.

Your next marker will be a fire hydrant on your right: opposite it is an opening between trees that leads to a gate. A sign tells you this is a Quaker cemetery, established in 1849—before the park was created. It remains property of the Society of Friends, so public access is prohibited. If it weren't, there would no doubt be a stream of visitors to the grave of movie star Montgomery Clift.

Resume walking on Center Drive, with the field known as the Nethermead on your right. At some point, move onto the path between the drive and the Nethermead, and take it to the end, where you see woods in front of you. Go left and walk under the Nethermead Arches, considered the geographic center of the park. There are three arches: one of them over the pedestrian lane you're on, one over a stream, and one above a bridle path.

Make the first right you can, which goes into the Ravine. Keep walking until you're on Rock Arch Bridge overlooking Ambergill Falls, then go up the steps to your right. Make a left and climb more steps; go to the right, and then to the right again. Cross Boulder Bridge and make a left.

Follow the trail, bypassing all turnoffs. When you reach the Y intersection with a tall tree in the triangle, go up the steps on the left. Continue along, and when you see the meadow, go to the left (walking with the meadow to your right). It dips back into the woods. When you can't go straight any farther and you see steps down on your left, go to the right. This trail will take you down several sets of steps on your way out of the Ravine.

Before heading to Long Meadow, take a moment to enjoy wooden Esdale Bridge and the cascading water beneath it to your left. Now turn around, and go left on the path beside the meadow. Cross Long Meadow at the next path, heading left when the path splits. Look out on the left for the Tennis House, designed by the same architects as the Boathouse in the same Palladian style. See it on all sides. The Tennis House was supposed to be a convenience for players of lawn tennis, a sport that was all the rage on Long Meadow when the building was conceived— but not so popular by the time it was completed.

Follow the path alongside West Drive in front of the Tennis House, walking with the Tennis House to your left. Turn right on the next cross path. To your left you should see the Bandshell, which in addition to other events hosts ❽ **Celebrate Brooklyn!,** a summer-long festival of rock, jazz, classical, reggae, funk, folk, Latino, and African concerts, as well as film screenings, dance, and family-oriented performances. Stay to the right (on the path next to the picnic tables), and when the path forks, go to the right and exit the park at 9th Street. The last monument on your walk is here: Daniel Chester French's bronze relief of the Marquis de Lafayette, depicted with his African horse groom.

Walk west on 9th for one block to the F/G trains.

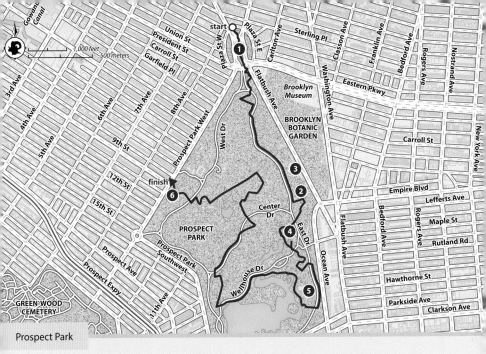

Prospect Park

Points of Interest

1 Grand Army Plaza (including Bailey Fountain and Soldiers' and Sailors' Memorial Arch) Flatbush Avenue and Vanderbilt Avenue; nycgovparks.org

2 **Lefferts Historic House** Near Flatbush Avenue and Empire Boulevard; 718-789-2822, historichousetrust.org/house/lefferts-historic-house-museum

3 **Prospect Park Zoo** Near Flatbush Avenue and Empire Boulevard; 718-399-7339, prospectparkzoo.com

4 **Audubon Center at the Boathouse** West of Ocean Avenue near Lincoln Road; 718-287-3400, ny.audubon.org/node/6906

5 **LeFrak Center at Lakeside** Off East Drive south of the Concert Grove; 718-462-0010, lakesidebrooklyn.com

6 **Celebrate Brooklyn!** Prospect Park Bandshell, off Prospect Park West and 10th Street; 718-683-5600, bricartsmedia.org/events-performances/bric-celebrate-brooklyn-festival

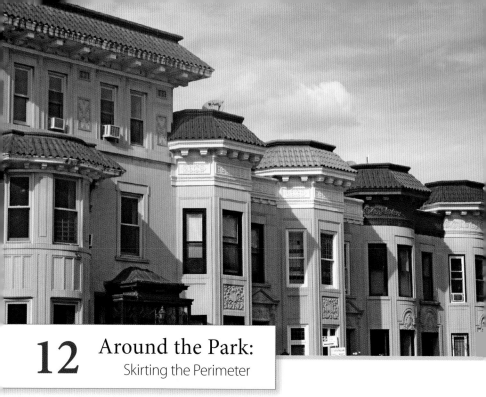

12 Around the Park:
Skirting the Perimeter

Above: These unusual and exuberant rowhouses on Maple Street in Prospect Lefferts Gardens were designed by architect Axel Hedman, who's also represented in Crown Heights

BOUNDARIES: Montgomery St., Rogers Ave., Parade Ground, 8th Ave.
DISTANCE: 5.2 miles
SUBWAY: F or G to 15th St. (Prospect Park W. exit)

Yes, yes, we know the shortest distance is always a straight line, but this walk from the westernmost to easternmost point of Prospect Park meanders deliberately. You go only a few steps into the park itself. Instead, the route takes you through some of the areas skirting the park, from Windsor Terrace south to the Parade Ground, then north through Prospect Lefferts Gardens to the Botanic Garden. (Park Slope and Prospect Heights, the other neighborhoods bordering the park, get their own walks.) One of the last stops on the walk is the most hallowed place in this city of churches—the site of Ebbets Field. It's been an apartment complex for more than 50 years but still exerts an emotional pull on baseball fans, Brooklyn nostalgists, and, perhaps, anyone who's ever had their heart broken.

Walk Description

In the subway, follow signs for Prospect Park West and go up the first staircase on your right to exit the station. You'll be facing a 1928 theater that at press time was being transformed into a seven-screen ❶ **Nitehawk Cinema,** specializing in themed and art-house programming and offering food and drink service at your seat, with menus specially crafted to accompany particular films.

Walk west—away from the park—on 14th Street. Some call this area South Slope, as opposed to Park Slope on the other side of 10th Street, although the distinction has been disappearing along with South Slope's affordability. This block is pure Park Slope in style, anyway, from the elegant Montauk apartment house on the right corner to the late-19th-century rowhouses.

Go right on 8th Avenue, but only for half a block, to check out stately P.S. 107 (1894). Then head in the other direction on 8th Avenue, past the fine-looking Park Slope Jewish Center (1925), and your attention is sure to be seized by the 14th Regiment Armory, erected in 1895. Don't miss what's to the right of the front door.

Make a left on 15th Street and proceed into Bartel-Pritchard Square, a circle centered on a black granite war memorial. Bartel and Pritchard were the surnames of two Brooklyn boys killed in World War I. Opposite, two columns designed by Stanford White gird the entrance to Prospect Park. Those urns atop them used to be lit nightly.

Walk away from the park on Prospect Park West. You are now in Windsor Terrace, traditionally home to many police officers and firefighters. Windsor Terrace native Vincent E. Brunton, for whom 16th Street is now named, was an FDNY captain who died in the World Trade Center collapse. He moonlighted as a bartender at ❷ **Farrell's,** the saloon on your left at 16th that's said to be one of the first bars to have opened in Brooklyn after Prohibition was repealed. Farrell's is famous for serving beer in giant Styrofoam cups (and for not serving unchaperoned women until the '70s). Hollywood has come calling repeatedly around here: Farrell's was featured in a scene with Helen Hunt and Shirley Knight in the Oscar-winning film *As Good As It Gets;* the corner across 16th is where Harvey Keitel had a shop in *Smoke;* and *Dog Day Afternoon* was filmed at a warehouse on Prospect Park West between 17th and 18th Streets that's been converted into condos.

Turn left on Windsor Place. Make a right on Howard Place, left on Prospect Avenue, and left on Fuller Place. The rowhouses on Howard and Fuller don't have the same pedigree as Park Slope's, but they certainly have their own charms (and porches!).

Turn right on Windsor Place. Sci-fi author Isaac Asimov lived on this block as a teenager in the 1930s; his parents owned a candy store at #174, and the family's apartment was across the street.

Make a right on 11th Avenue.

Go left on Prospect Avenue. After the Seeley Street overpass, observe the ❸ **organic vegetable farm** that residents have created. Across Vanderbilt Street, a number of restaurants have sprung up in just the past few years. Past Greenwood Avenue, the limestone-and-brick firehouse on the left was constructed in 1896 and originally manned by volunteers, who watched for fires from that picturesque tower.

Turn around and go right on Greenwood Avenue. An assortment of interesting houses, generally from the early 1900s, are clustered around East 7th Street and the block to Sherman Street. Continue to Prospect Park Southwest, cross to the park side, and make a right. You will walk around a colonnaded pavilion, one of a pair of public-transit shelters near this park entrance that were designed by Stanford White in 1896. Passengers could sit on a marble bench and stare up at a floral embossed ceiling while waiting for the horsecar. The dramatic *Horse Tamers* sculptures flanking this entrance were unveiled in 1899. The artist was Frederick MacMonnies, who did several pieces for the park.

Cross Parkside Avenue at the second shelter. Walk along Park Circle, with the tennis center on your left, then go left on Coney Island Avenue.

Make a left at the Bowling Green gate to the ❹ **Parade Ground.** You can see to your right where early park users played lawn bowling; now it has a riding ring and corral for horses. (Kensington Stables, est. 1930, the sole remaining stable for Prospect Park riders, is off Coney Island Avenue on Caton Place.) Created at the same time as the park, the Parade Ground was designed for the staging of military pageants but has provided many more years of service to athletics than the military. Stay on the path until you have a soccer field in front of you, and make a left. Then take a right on the path between baseball diamonds. Future major leaguers Sandy Koufax, Joe Torre, Willie Randolph, and Manny Ramirez were all scouted by the pros while playing at the Parade Ground.

Turn left at the snack bar, then make a right when you reach Parkside Avenue. Watch on your left for the colonnaded structure on elevated ground within the park, and go up to it. Officially it's a peristyle, as seen in classical Greek architecture, but it is also referred to as the Grecian Shelter and was originally used as a viewing promontory for Parade Ground events. The design, if not the upkeep, is magnificent (thank Stanford White): limestone columns, glazed brick floor, Guastavino tile ceiling.

Back on Parkside, continue east and turn right onto Parade Place. Then make a left on Crooke Avenue. Note the pretty rowhouses, amply set back from the sidewalk, on your left as you cross St. Paul Place. Continue on Crooke past a series of detached houses on your right.

Turn left on Ocean Avenue, one of Brooklyn's grand boulevards, known for its classic apartment buildings. Examine and admire the detail on #365, 361, 353, and 354.

At Parkside Avenue, with the so-called pergola entrance to Prospect Park on your left, make a right.

Turn left on Flatbush Avenue. You're now in the neighborhood of Prospect Lefferts Gardens, which grew out of a development named Lefferts Manor. In the 1890s, with the new Prospect Park an attractive local amenity and the even newer Brooklyn Bridge easing the commute to Manhattan, communities developed around Flatbush. Lefferts Manor was initiated by a member of the Lefferts family who'd been farming this land since 1660. He divided his property into 600 lots and established covenants for those building homes: among other restrictions, they had to be single-family houses, set back from the street at least 14 feet. Construction continued into the 1920s.

Turn right on Fenimore Street. The earliest houses within the original Lefferts Manor community are #107 and #115, both built in 1896. These and the other freestanding houses on the block are wood-frame structures, which actually contradicted the Lefferts rule for property buyers that houses be made of brick or stone.

Turn left on Bedford Avenue, then left on Rutland Road. Much of the right side flanking the green-shuttered brick houses dates from Lefferts Manor's first wave of construction. Then you have a row of houses on each side that combine Tudor fronts with Spanish-tile roofs. Note that every other one has an angled bay window and rectangular door and first-floor windows . . . or a flat bay and arched openings on the ground floor. These are identical to what you find on Chester Court, a cul-de-sac off Flatbush Avenue that earned historic-district designation. The ones here on Rutland were built a few years later, in 1914–15.

Turn right on Flatbush, then right on Midwood Street. The facing rows of #51–71 and #52–72 were the first homes offered by William A. A. Brown, Lefferts Manor's most prolific developer in its early years. These are from 1898 and are identical but in the opposite order, so the first house you pass on the right will match the last in the row on the left.

Make a left on Bedford and a right on Maple Street, a visually striking block thanks to those multicolored Spanish-tile roofs sitting atop the bays like wide-brimmed hats.

Turn left on Rogers Avenue and then left on Lincoln Road. At Bedford Avenue, ❺ **Grace Reformed Church** (1893) makes a cute picture with its terra cotta trim and cone-shaped tower roof. Turn right on Bedford.

At Empire Boulevard, you cross into Crown Heights. Proceed toward the massive and foreboding high-rises at Sullivan Place. This is what's become of Ebbets Field, ballpark of the Brooklyn Dodgers—a team that captured the hearts and minds of fans like no other team in any sport, that put an end to the ban on black players, that made up for years of agony with a World Series victory over the Yankees in 1955, and that two years later was packed up and taken to Los Angeles by owner Walter O'Malley, who would be reviled in Brooklyn for generations. These apartments have now been here longer than Ebbets Field was (1913–1960). Continue up Bedford, which aligned with the right-field wall.

Turn left on Montgomery Street, flanked by two schools named for civil rights icons. Medgar Evers College is on your right; Jackie Robinson School, a public elementary school, is down McKeever Place to your left. At Franklin Avenue, look past the smokestack at the brick building with the "witch's hat" dormers.

Turn left on Franklin. Smell spices? Morris J. Golombeck, a fourth-generation spice maker and importer, has used these facilities since 1955. Past the loading dock, look between the windows of those triple arches for beer barrels sculpted in the ledge. This complex—including the structures on Montgomery—was built for the Consumers Park brewery, later renamed Interboro. It also had a beer garden, restaurant, hotel, and concert stage on the premises, but a little something called Prohibition put an end to it all.

Back at Empire Boulevard, go right. The red-roofed building on the right belongs to the fire department; it was the Brooklyn dispatch center from 1913 to 2008, and was granted landmark status for being such an alluring utilitarian structure.

At Flatbush Avenue is an entry gate for the ❻ Brooklyn Botanic Garden, where our walk concludes. Its Japanese garden, featuring a pond, wooden bridges, and Shinto shrine, is many New Yorkers' favorite place to escape the frenetic urban pace. The 52-acre Botanic Garden also contains Brooklyn's version of the Hollywood Walk of Fame—a path of stones inscribed with names of famous Brooklynites. Other highlights include herb, rock, and rose gardens, a scenic overlook, a large greenhouse, a bonsai museum, a lily-pad reflecting pool, and cherry trees. In all, about 18,000 plant varieties are found within the garden, which has welcomed guests since 1911.

From this Botanic Garden gate, walk south on Flatbush or Ocean Avenue approximately three blocks to Lincoln Road for the B, Q, or S.

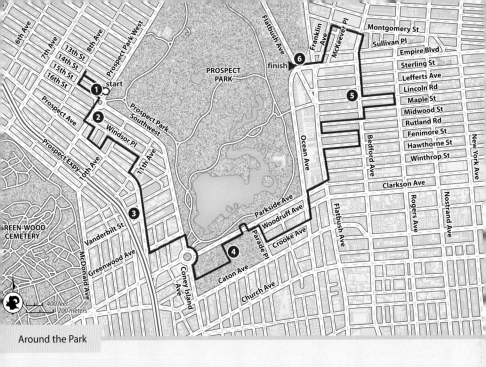

Points of Interest

1. **Nitehawk Cinema** 188 Prospect Park W.; 718-782-8370, nitehawkcinema.com
2. **Farrell's** 215 Prospect Park W.; 718-788-8779
3. **Prospect Farm** 1194 Prospect Ave.; prospectfarm.org
4. **Parade Ground** Parkside Avenue and Coney Island Avenue; 718-438-3435, nycgovparks.org
5. **Grace Reformed Church** 1800 Bedford Ave.; 718-287-4343, facebook.com/pg/GRCBrooklyn
6. **Brooklyn Botanic Garden** 1000 Washington Ave.; 718-623-7200, bbg.org

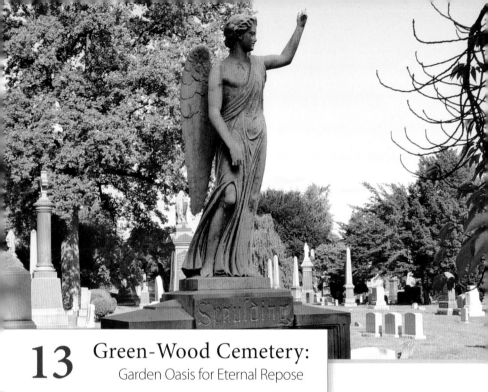

13 Green-Wood Cemetery:
Garden Oasis for Eternal Repose

Above: Green-Wood could also be considered a sculpture park or arboretum

BOUNDARIES: 4th Ave., 20th St., Fort Hamilton Pkwy., 36th St. (outside the cemetery)
DISTANCE: Approx. 7.5 miles
SUBWAY: R to 25th St.

Dead men—and women—tell a lot of tales at Green-Wood. They are tales of life in 19th-century New York, tales of the Civil War, tales of fame and infamy, tales of fortunes made, art created, companies and cities built, of causes championed, tragedies endured, and firsts accomplished. Since it opened in 1840, more than 550,000 people have been laid to rest at Green-Wood, one of the nation's first cemeteries not located within a churchyard. Some of its "permanent residents" are still well known today, others were prominent in their day but since forgotten, and plenty were ordinary citizens. But focusing strictly on the deceased is missing the point, and beauty, of Green-Wood. This 478-acre greensward of hills and ponds was designed to be a rural oasis in a harsh industrialized city. There were almost no public parks when it opened, so people came here to reconnect with nature and enjoy the outdoors. It contains a fascinating collection of statuary, too. In the mid-1800s, Green-Wood was the nation's top tourist attraction after Niagara Falls. In the 2000s, expanded hours, outreach, and special-event programming have restored it as a park and sightseeing destination.

Note: You can do half of this walk if you're not up for all of it, by either beginning or ending at Green-Wood's entrance on Fort Hamilton Parkway—just off the intersection within the cemetery of Border and Vine Avenues. Either wrap up or start your walk near Charles Feltman's grave (not quite the midpoint, about 4.2 miles into the walk). Just be aware that as of early 2017, the Fort Hamilton entrance was open only on weekends. The nearest subway is the F/G's Fort Hamilton Parkway station, roughly six blocks east.

Walk Description

From the subway, walk up 25th Street to 5th Avenue. Before crossing 5th to the cemetery entrance, note the landmarked ❶ **Weir Greenhouse** on your right. Green-Wood is restoring this 1895 structure—the only extant Victorian commercial greenhouse in the city—and incorporating it into a new visitor center.

Cross the avenue and enter through Richard Upjohn's Gothic brownstone gates, which feature sandstone reliefs of death and resurrection. You may hear squawking coming from the gates, or see birds flying in and out of the peaks. These are green parakeets from South America that started nesting here after they broke out of their crate at the airport in 1980. Or so the story goes. Go to the right, on Landscape Avenue, and walk toward the ❷ **chapel.** As you approach the oval in front of the chapel, look on your right for an old hitching post—a relic from the days when people traveled to Green-Wood by horse-drawn carriage. The chapel was modeled on Christ Church in Oxford, England, and designed in 1911 by the architects of Grand Central Terminal. It's open to the public when no services are being conducted inside.

With your back to the chapel, go left up the ramp to Landscape Avenue, where you can see a strangely sensual male angel, large wings rising high above his head. Turn left on Landscape, cross Valley Avenue, and make a left on Ridge Path. Past a large tree on your right, next to the Nash obelisk, the lamb sculpture at the Hickson grave is eroding. Lambs are a common motif on children's graves, symbolizing their innocence. Other recurring sights in Green-Wood include draped urns—symbolizing what is left on earth after the soul ascends to heaven (the urn represents the body, or container of the soul; the shroud, the cover of the casket)—and spheres, symbolizing eternity.

Go onto the grass to your left from the path and walk past two crosses to the plain graves of two men who brought much sparkle and dazzle into the world: Charles Lewis Tiffany, founder of the jewelry store that bears his name, and his son Louis Comfort, the stained-glass artist who made windows and lamps.

Go down Vale Path next to the Tiffany graves and turn left on Valley Avenue. Walk with the water to your right. Turn left at Dew Path, then right on Hillside Path. Asher Durand, Hudson River School painter, is buried on your left, behind the Woodmans, his daughter's in-laws. Durand's masterpiece, *Kindred Spirits,* was sold in 2005 for $35 million, then a record for an American painting.

Follow Hillside to the right back to Valley, where you can't miss the ornate tomb of John Matthews on your left. Matthews, known as the "soda fountain king" for his invention of machines that carbonated and dispensed beverages, is the man looking up at a ceiling that depicts events in his life. The seated figure above symbolizes grief.

Walk downhill on Walnut Avenue and make a left at Lake Avenue. On your left, a woman with flowers stands over the grave of George Tilyou, the Coney Island legend who created its great amusement park Steeplechase. Continue on Lake past the grove of bushes on your right. Turn right on Sylvan Avenue and look in the island on your left for the grave of Do-Hum-Me, an American Indian chief's daughter who became a star attraction of P. T. Barnum shows.

Proceed on Sylvan Avenue past the Sylvan Water on your left. Just before the next fork, find D. R. Bennett's grave. Bennett, a Shaker-turned-freethinker, was jailed for mailing out his anti-religion tracts—in violation of the anti-obscenity Comstock laws. As you can tell from his verbose grave, he couldn't have been an easy person to muzzle.

Turn left on Spruce Avenue. Then go left on Anemone Path and right on Ridge Path. Stay to the right when the path diverges. One of the tombs along the pond that you're overlooking contains songwriter Fred Ebb, who penned the lyrics to *Cabaret, Chicago,* and "New York, New York."

Go left onto Cedar Path, then left on Lake Avenue. Take Ravine Path on your right up and over to Oak Avenue, where you should make a left. Crusading newspaperman Horace Greeley is buried on a hill to your left. Despite his oft-quoted advice, the bust of him does not face west. You can spot it from the avenue, but you'll have to climb if you want to see the bas-relief images of his profession (man at printing press, quill pen and paper, and so on) on his monument.

Across Oak Avenue from Greeley, go on Winterberry Path to a big, knobby tree. Go left to the angel of death weeping over the Cassard grave. Several 9/11 casualties are buried in this area, including firefighters Cherry, Agnello, and Vega in a cluster directly across from Greeley. About 75 people who died in the terrorist attacks are buried at Green-Wood.

With your back to Greeley's grave, go down the lawn to Landscape Avenue and make a right. Turn left on Circling Path, then take the path to the right of the tree. Between two tall trees on your right, there's a statue of a man with a doting young woman—the GRANDPA AND HIS LOVING GRANDDAUGHTER, who are buried together.

Go back on Circling Path and continue in the direction you'd been headed. Turn left when you reach the avenue. As it curves around, you'll find the largest mausoleum in Green-Wood, constructed in the 1870s for the Steinways, piano makers extraordinaire, by John Moffitt, sculptor of the reliefs on the brownstone entrance gates. It cost almost $2 million in today's dollars and contains 119 rooms, though fewer than 60 Steinways ended up here. Continue around the oval to Thorn Path and go left. Cross Highwood and walk up the lawn to the tall monument shaped like a concave triangle. Telegraph inventor Samuel Morse is buried here with his brothers. Take Highwood down to Orchard Avenue and go left.

Walking on Orchard, pass Tulip Path and watch on the right for a big tree at the avenue's edge. Next to it, firefighter George Kerr's grave shows his helmet, ax, and hose—one of several Green-Wood monuments honoring the fire department. Another profession well represented in the cemetery is baseball. The game's first superstar, James Creighton Jr., is buried on your right. Baseball bats are carved down the sides of his grave and within the wreath, along with a ball, base, and scorebook. Creighton was a fearsome pitcher *and* slugger who died at age 21 of a ruptured bladder, said to be caused by his swinging too hard at the baseball.

Follow Orchard downhill, then go left on Crescent Avenue, walking beside Dell Water and then Crescent Water. Go onto Dale Avenue, then right on Vernal Avenue. Turn left at Union Avenue, then right on Southwood. Stay to the left as the road curves and becomes Locust Avenue.

Go right on Violet Path, then right on Circlet. On your right you'll pass the grave of James Merritt Ives, printer of iconic pictures of wintertime idylls. Keep walking around Circlet to Fir Path and make a left, then a right on Vista Avenue. After Southwood, this will take you onto Grape Avenue. At its intersection with Locust, two stone posts to your left identify a ❸ Roosevelt plot. Among those buried here are Martha and Alice Roosevelt, the mother and first wife of Teddy Roosevelt. He was serving in the New York State Assembly—his first public office—when he rushed home after his wife took ill following childbirth. Upon arrival, he discovered that his mother's cold had escalated to typhoid. The women died in the same house on the same day in 1884.

Across Grape from the Roosevelts, follow Hazel Path all the way to Vernal Avenue and turn right. Watch on your left for the Moorish mausoleum of industrialist Cornelius Garrison, 1853–54 mayor of San Francisco who later moved to New York and headed shipping and rail concerns.

Walk up Jonquil Path behind Garrison's mausoleum and turn right on Cypress Avenue. Then go left on Dale. Turn right on Sassafras Avenue to see the enormous sword-bearing angel sitting on the Rinelli Guardino mausoleum. Then go back on Sassafras—a playful name that doesn't prepare you for the startling image coming up after you turn right on Dale: a bride reclining beneath the cross of the Merello Volta grave. Little is known about the deceased, but unconfirmed rumors say she was a Mob bride whacked on her wedding day. Brace yourself for another creepy sculpture after you turn left from Dale onto Fir Avenue. (Before you reach it, you can detour left on Mistletoe Path and look amid the row of simple, low-lying graves to your right for artist Jean-Michel Basquiat.) To your left on Fir is another representation of the angel of death—a cloak without a body inside. It marks the grave of Charles and Mary Schieren, who died a day apart in 1915. He was a former mayor of Brooklyn.

Cross Grape Avenue, and turn right from Fir onto Vine Avenue, lined with all kinds of intriguing statuary. Turn left on Border, whose extravagant burial sites include the tomb of Charles Feltman, with cupola and angel on top. Feltman was a Coney Island restaurateur who came up with the idea to put a sausage in a bun for eating without silverware . . . and the hot dog was born.

Continue on Border to the ❹ Hillside Mausoleum at Cypress Avenue, where you can take a break. This 21st-century addition to Green-Wood features a five-story atrium, pyramid skylights, reflecting pools, and Tibetan wool carpets.

Exit the mausoleum on level 3, onto Dawn Path. On your right is the squat, plain grave of celebrity clergyman and liberal firebrand Henry Ward Beecher, who preached in Brooklyn Heights for nearly 40 years. He lies with his wife; his mistress, Elizabeth Tilton, is buried elsewhere in Green-Wood. Throughout the rabidly publicized scandal of their affair, Beecher refused to acknowledge he had behaved immorally, and his epitaph indicates he took that conviction to the grave.

Head down Dawn, and at the intersection with Hillside is the pyramid tomb of Henry Bergh, founder of the American Society for the Prevention of Cruelty to Animals (ASPCA).

Go right on Hillside. Inside the churchlike mausoleum adorned with bronze statues on your left at Ocean Avenue, John Mackay and his wife were laid to rest in a heated marble tomb that contains an altar and pietà and was wired for electric lighting. With the Mackays to your left, walk on Ocean. Make the first right onto Atlantic Avenue and follow it to a loop. Halfway around, go onto Grove Avenue to your left, then right onto Central Avenue. Stay on Central to the next avenue where you can go right. Take that to Atlantic Avenue and make a left.

Watch for the Badger and Wilcox monuments on your right. Look about four rows behind them to a statue of a drummer boy. This is the grave of Clarence Mackenzie, a 12-year-old regiment drummer who was the first Brooklynite to give his life in the Civil War. Many Civil War veterans are buried in this area, as well as a 19th-century artist named William Beard. You shouldn't have any trouble finding his grave a little farther along on Atlantic, as it's guarded by his favorite subject—the bear. (He often painted them dancing.)

Follow Atlantic onto Meadow, then back onto Atlantic. Turn left on Hydrangea Path and watch immediately for the Griffith grave. On the side facing away from Hydrangea, husband Charles had his last memory of JANE MY WIFE sculpted in marble: saying goodbye to him outside their Greenwich Village townhouse (see his carriage over on the right). She died unexpectedly of heart failure while he was at work.

Continue on Hydrangea to Fern Avenue and make a left. On your left at Greenbough Avenue, an elaborate altar with weeping angels memorializes 17-year-old Charlotte Canda. The only child of a Napoleonic officer who had immigrated to New York, Charlotte was killed when she was thrown from a carriage after the horses pulling it were startled by a storm.

Go right on Greenbough. A gray obelisk on a hill to your right, behind two crosses, marks the grave of Henry Raymond, founder of *The New York Times*. He also cofounded the Republican Party, which might surprise some present-day Republicans. Walk slightly downhill to your right to the intersection with Sycamore Avenue. On your left, Rex the dog sits, appropriately, beside a tree. Stay on Greenbough, making a left at the next fork and then another quick left.

Turn right onto Myrtle Path and ascend to the ❺ **Pierreponts' hill** and the Gothic Revival brownstone structure (by Richard Upjohn) that's been described as an "open-air church." Henry Pierrepont was involved in the creation of Green-Wood and in the planning of Brooklyn's streets; his father was a major landowner in early Brooklyn, and his great-grandfather cofounded Yale.

Go back down Myrtle and turn left. Follow the road (Central Avenue) straight and turn right onto Bayside Avenue. Turn right on Blossom Path, following it to your left at the Simmons grave. Go to your right when you reach the avenue, then turn left on Rue Path. Continue uphill when another path crosses it, then go straight onto Bay Grove Path and follow it as it winds its way down to the oval dominated by the bronze statue of ❻ **DeWitt Clinton.** Before Clinton, you'll pass the grave of printmaker Nathaniel Currier, buried with his two wives and infant children. DeWitt Clinton—mayor of New York City, governor of New York State, US Senator, and runner-up to James Madison in the 1812 presidential election—was buried in the state capital of Albany upon his death in 1828, and his 1853 reinterment at Green-Wood was a masterstroke of publicity for the fledgling cemetery. Clinton's pedestal exhibits scenes from the development of the Erie Canal, which he spearheaded.

Walk up Bayside Path behind Clinton's grave, taking note to your right as you get on the path of "Little Frankie," the statue of a child that was crafted by Daniel Chester French, who sculpted Lincoln for the Lincoln Memorial. Turn right and then quickly left on Highland Avenue.

Make a left at Fern Avenue. Go up the second staircase on your right to the Pilot's Monument, erected at the grave of ship pilot Thomas Freeborn, who perished when his vessel was battered by a storm. The incident is depicted on the sarcophagus, and above it a mast with its top cut off alludes to Freeborn's premature death. Fittingly, this spot offers a superb view across the harbor.

From Fern Avenue, turn right on Mulberry Avenue, then left on Hemlock Avenue. On your left at the intersection with Battle Avenue, the bust on a pedestal marks the grave of Elias Howe Jr., inventor of the sewing machine. Behind the bust is the grave of pet Fannie, inscribed with a poem countering those who might question the fuss over "only a dog" (the opening words). Proceed on Hemlock across Battle Avenue and take the first path on the right. Then go left onto Coronilla Path.

Turn right on Garland Avenue. You will approach the gigantic ❼ *Civic Virtue* statue from behind. It was this rear view from his office in City Hall, in fact, that Mayor Fiorello La Guardia objected to—so much so that he sent the statue to Queens, where it stood in front of Borough Hall on Queens Boulevard from 1941 to 2011. Public opinion turned against it over the years because of its depiction of the man seemingly trampling on women (who represent vice). The parents and brother of the sculptor, Frederick MacMonnies, are buried in Green-Wood.

Facing Mr. Virtue, go to the right, onto Jasmine Avenue. Then turn left on Border Avenue. Watch on your right for the Ricke grave and go behind it to Henry Chadwick, the so-called Father of Baseball. A member of the Baseball Hall of Fame, Chadwick invented the box score and scoring system, as well as much of baseball's terminology, from *single, left on base,* and *double play* to the slangier *goose egg* and *chin music*. His monument features a large baseball on top, and bronze renderings of bats, a glove, and a catcher's mask affixed to its sides. A mini baseball diamond with granite "bases" lies before the grave.

Continue on Border to the nearby intersection with Hemlock Avenue. On your left lies Clara Ruppertz. Read the tablet held by the life-size female figure to learn what Clara's kin thought of her.

Go onto Hemlock Avenue. Mere steps in on your right you'll see the decorous resting place of John Torrio, which belies his conduct in life: he ran Chicago's prostitution and bootlegging rackets before Al Capone. He's the rare capo to die of natural causes (a heart attack). Other gangsters buried in Green-Wood who died from more conventional causes include Albert Anastasia, who was shot to death while getting a haircut in a barbershop, and "Crazy Joe" Gallo, gunned down during his birthday dinner at a Little Italy restaurant.

Farther along Hemlock, to your right behind the Seamans tomb, sits the modest grave of Juan Trippe, founder of Pan Am Airways. Turn right on Garland Avenue. Before you turn left on Battle Path, look up the hill opposite it at the grave of Charles H. Ebbets, owner of the Brooklyn Dodgers. Then take Battle Path to the bronze statue of Minerva, the Roman goddess of battle, at the ❽ **Altar of Liberty**—a tribute to the Battle of Brooklyn, which was fought on this hill. Charles Higgins, an ink and adhesive magnate (who's buried behind Minerva), commissioned the monument for the

144th anniversary of the battle in 1920. It was positioned so Liberty is waving to Liberty—if you haven't already noticed the lady in the harbor, just turn around when you're in front of Minerva.

Turn left on Liberty Path and look to your right for the in-ground gravestone of legendary composer and conductor Leonard Bernstein. Visitors usually leave stones on the grave—a way of paying respect to the dead in Judaism.

Go back to Battle Path and turn left. The Soldiers' Monument is a proud achievement of Green-Wood and one of the earliest Civil War memorials, erected in 1869. It honors the 148,000 New Yorkers who fought for the Union with statues of a cavalryman (with sword), engineer (ax), infantryman (gun), and artilleryman. They're on a hill that's the highest natural point in Brooklyn.

At Battle Avenue, across from Battle Hill, R. H. McDonald's headstone is crammed with a temperance diatribe that relegates his wife, Sarah, to a corner—though her family ties (see what it says) may have been more worthy of note. Facing this grave, go right on Battle Avenue, which promptly curves to the left.

To your right at Bayview Avenue, a Sphinx guards a pyramid, its doorway flanked by Jesus and Mary. Albert Parsons, a fan of Egyptiana who wrote a book about the Pyramids, is entombed here. Adding to the religious mix, a sculpture of Moses and his mother sits on a gravestone to the left. Proceed on Battle to the Greek-temple-style tomb of tobacco mogul John Anderson. If you walk on the grass behind Anderson, you'll come to Frederick A. O. Schwarz, namesake of the toy emporium.

Across Battle Avenue from John Anderson, go on Bayview Path, and don't turn till you reach Bayview Avenue. You need take only a few steps to your right to behold the gravesite of Louis Moreau Gottschalk, a famed concert pianist and the first internationally renowned American classical composer. Gottschalk was conducting a performance of his work in Brazil when he died at age 40 in 1869. The charming bronze angel, who's cupping her ear to hear music, was unveiled in 2012 after Green-Wood held a design competition to bring a sculpture back to Gottschalk's grave. Its original marble angel had been destroyed by vandals in 1959.

Facing Gottschalk, go to your right on Bayview Avenue. When you reach Battle, a memorial stands on your left to those lost in the Brooklyn Theater fire of 1876. The fire broke out backstage just as the play was ending and quickly spread throughout the theater, claiming 278 lives.

Turn right on Battle Avenue, heading back toward the brownstone entry gates. On your left at Arbor Avenue, note the serene angels sculpted in bronze on the Stewart mausoleum, as well as the cherub faces along the top. They are the work of sculptor Augustus Saint-Gaudens, and the tomb itself was designed by architect Stanford White. The Stewarts were the parents of Isabella Stewart Gardner, whose private collection became Boston's premier art museum.

Follow Battle back to the main gates, one block from the R train at 25th and 4th.

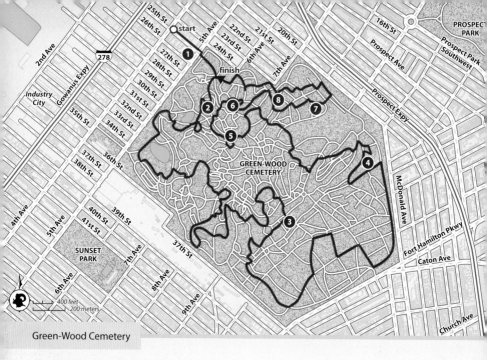

Green-Wood Cemetery

Points of Interest

1 **Weir Greenhouse** 25th Street and 5th Avenue

2 **Chapel** Landscape and Battle Avenues

3 **Roosevelts** Locust and Grape Avenues

4 **Hillside Mausoleum** Border and Cypress Avenues

5 **Pierreponts** Myrtle Path off Central Avenue

6 **DeWitt Clinton** Bayside Avenue and Bay Grove Path

7 *Civic Virtue* Hemlock and Jasmine Avenues

8 **Battle Hill/Altar of Liberty** North of Border Avenue between Battle and Garland Avenues

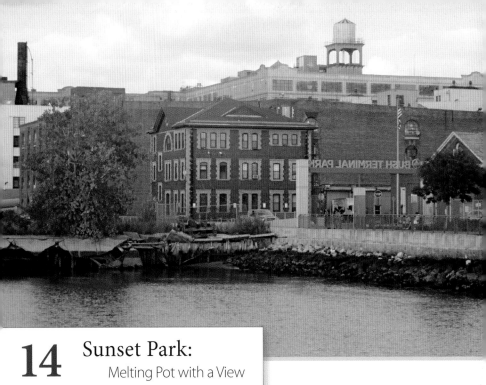

14 Sunset Park:
Melting Pot with a View

Above: Old Bush Terminal buildings, seen from waterside paths within the new Bush Terminal Park

BOUNDARIES: 35th St., 8th Ave., 62nd St., Bush Terminal Park
DISTANCE: 4.3 miles
SUBWAY: N to 8th Ave.

With the transformation of defunct Bush Terminal into the Industry City office and retail complex, Sunset Park got its own "city." But you'll also find the *world* within this polyglot neighborhood. Now brimming with Chinese, Latino, Turkish, and Southeast Asian residents, Sunset Park still bears influences from the Scandinavians, Irish, and other Europeans who lived here in past generations. Outside of its ethnic diversity, Sunset Park boasts a rich industrial heritage. The southern terminus of Brooklyn's commercial waterfront, it bustled with activity in the first half of the 20th century. After a period of decline, the area near the water has been reborn with food artisans, media and tech firms, and designers and manufacturers based at Industry City.

Walk Description

Upon leaving the train station, cross 8th Avenue and look down 62nd Street. You should be able to see the Norwegian flag and letters of SPORTING CLUB GJØA painted on the side of a building. The Norwegian Folk Dance Society of New York practices in that building, home base of a soccer club founded around 1912. With the subway station on your left, proceed on 8th Avenue into the heart of Brooklyn's Chinatown. But wait, that white steeple down 60th to your right is a Mormon church, and the United American Muslim Association is here on the right between 60th and 59th. And in another instance of Sunset Park's multiculti heritage, it's in a building that used to be an Irish dance club. Visitors are welcome: ❶ **Fatih Camii,** the mosque inside, is a vision in blue, with imported Turkish tiles adorning the walls.

The Chinese fish and seafood markets on 8th Avenue, while impressive in selection and price, can be unsettling for some sensibilities with their tanks of live animals—turtles, eels, and whole squid among them—to be bought and cooked. Mind your step: some of those crabs are frisky and jump out of the vats. Also watch out for the most humongous clams you've likely ever seen. Chinese businesses along 8th sell everything from insurance to toys, and plenty of edible and nonedible merchandise is hawked out on the sidewalks. There's also a Malaysian and Vietnamese presence. On your right at 52nd Street, the Second Evangelical Free Church was built in 1913 by Norwegians and now has a majority Indian congregation as well as a Chinese ministry.

Turn left on 49th, a street not dissimilar from its neighbors but allowed to use the more evocative coname Sunset Terrace.

Turn right at 7th Avenue, passing two century-old churches in succession on your right. They both serve Spanish-speaking parishioners, and enormous St. Agatha also has Chinese services. Across from Church of the Redeemer, ❷ **Helado de Coco** is a favorite place to cool off in summer with a tropical-flavored ice or ice cream. Sunset Park's Latino population started with Puerto Ricans arriving in the 1950s, but nowadays more residents come from Mexico, Ecuador, the Dominican Republic, and Central America. A Buddhist temple adds a pop of color between 46th and 45th. On your left across 45th, Christ United Methodist is another church with Norwegian roots.

Turn right on 44th Street, a hub of what used to be called Finntown. The two churches on this block were originally, on your left, Finnish Golgotha Congregational and farther down on your right, Finnish Evangelical Lutheran.

Make a left on 8th Avenue, then a right on 43rd Street and go to the second apartment house on your right. It says ALKU TOINEN—that is, Alku No. 2, the first Alku (Finnish for "beginning") being the adjacent building. These were New York City's first-ever nonprofit cooperative apartments, their construction costs paid for by the families that would live there (plus loans from both the bank and neighbors who got behind this socialist concept). They opened in 1916, and within a decade Finns had built more than 25 others in the neighborhood.

Turn around and head west on 43rd. At 7th Avenue, cross over, go right and take the steps up into Sunset Park. If the recreation center is open, go inside to see historic photos as well as the Art Deco ticket booth, locker-room signs, floor tiles, and ceiling light fixtures. The building *and* pool are designated city landmarks, created by the WPA in 1936.

Facing the rec center, go to your right—appreciate the building's exterior brickwork as you pass—then stay to the left when the path splits. Continue past the basketball courts to the flag-pole, which was erected after the park's carousel was removed. It is remembered with imprints of carousel horses in the pavement. The long four-story apartment buildings across from the park on 41st Street were built as Finnish nonprofit co-ops in the 1920s. Wander around the park as much as you'd like. Sitting as it does on a 200-foot-high hill, the park offers sweeping views of the harbor, the Statue of Liberty, the Manhattan skyline, and Brooklyn's own skyscrapers.

Leave the park on 5th Avenue at 43rd Street via the grand staircase with masonry urns at top and bottom. Go straight down 43rd. The former courthouse on your right at 4th Avenue was designed in 1931 by an architect who'd had a hand in Grand Central Terminal. Diagonally across from it is perhaps the saddest orphan in New York City architecture. This Romanesque "castle," built in 1886 for a police precinct and stable, has been vacant since the 1970s. It's had a series of owners with unrealized plans, and the latest reports have the board of education looking to con-vert it to a public school. Whatever condition you find it in, it deserves admirers, what with those busts, terra cotta moldings, ironwork fleurs-de-lis, Venetian-style arcade, and so forth.

Facing the castle, go to the right on 4th Avenue. St. Michael's, the church whose cupola-topped 200-foot tower was visible from the park, extends nearly to 3rd Avenue. Also take a look at the 42nd Street side of the former courthouse opposite the church.

From 4th Avenue, turn left on 40th Street.

Cross 3rd Avenue and go to the right, passing in front of Frankel's, which opened as a sort of general store for dockworkers in 1890. It's one of the few retailers to survive the construction of the Gowanus Expressway in the 1940s. Before then, 3rd Avenue was a social and commercial heart of Sunset Park. A thousand people lost their homes so the highway could be built, and it created a rupture between industrial and residential districts. On the next block, as you walk alongside the Costco parking lot, you get your first good view of a building of ❹ **Industry City.** When this was Bush Terminal, 25 shipping lines used its 18 piers and 22-block spread of warehouses, which had been considered a boondoggle when oil scion Irving T. Bush conceived it in 1890.

Make a left on 37th Street. Go into #241 to begin your trip through "Innovation Alley," the north–south passage running through the buildings of Industry City. Come out the other side and enjoy the courtyard, which has a performance stage at the east end.

Go into the next building for the food hall and walk through it in both directions—not just to get something to eat but to watch the vittles being made. At the east end of the food hall (to your right upon entering) is an art gallery; at the west end, check out the Landing, an enormous rec room with shabby-chic furniture, nautical-themed sculpture, and foosball, Nok Hockey, and billiards tables. Adjacent to it is a store that sells items made at Industry City.

Cross 36th Street and go through the next building. From the courtyard, enter Building 4 toward the east to find ❺ **Li-Lac Chocolates.** Samples are given in the store, and next to it, you'll have visions of *I Love Lucy* looking at the bonbon assembly line. Exit onto 35th Street and readjust your taste buds as you cross the street to Brooklyn Brine Co., whose pickles come in such varieties as Maple Bourbon and Damn Spicy. Near the center of this building, visit the Extraction Lab, a café where baristas brew coffee and tea on $14,000 "Steampunk" machines operated via an iPad app—and you can pay up to $18 for a cup! Farther west in this building, go upstairs for the ❻ **Industry City Distillery,** makers of vodka who open for tastings and tours on weekends. From here you can head to 2nd Avenue and go left (walking with these buildings on your left), or first explore more of Industry City and its continually expanding array of artisans and specialty vendors.

Proceed south on 2nd Avenue. Those tracks are remnants of the dedicated railroad that served Bush Terminal, which also had its own power plant, police force, and fire department.

Turn right on 42nd Street, a block bookended by distinctive architecture. First there's that terra cotta bell capping the corner building on your right. Then, nearing 1st Avenue on your left, is a medieval fortress of a warehouse, built in 1890 and studded with what look like cast-iron mandalas.

Turn left on 1st Avenue and see the warehouse's Gothic tower, set back from the street.

Make a right at 43rd Street, walking between the brick pillars and then straight ahead until you're standing before Mr. Bush himself—in copper-statue form above the onetime entrance to his offices. The large buildings to your right have been earmarked for a "Made in NY" campus for garment manufacturing and film and TV production, announced in early 2017.

Go to the left toward the ❽ **Bush Terminal Park** gate. Enter the park for an incredible change of scenery. Roam the jetties, gaze into the tidal pools, follow the paved path up and around the woodsy hillock, find that scenic nook in its south corner. Or just park yourself on a bench or boulder and take in the views; obviously, the skyline steals focus, but do a 360-degree scan.

That's the end of the tour, but you have to walk to 3rd Avenue or 39th Street for a bus. The nearest subway station is on 4th Avenue at 45th Street.

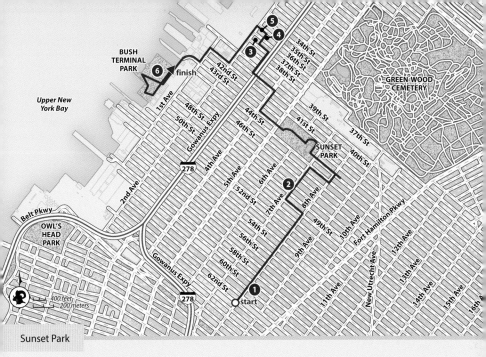

Points of Interest

1. **Fatih Camii** 5911 8th Ave.; 718-438-6919

2. **Helado de Coco** 4716 7th Ave.; 347-987-3958, luvums.com

3. **Industry City** 2nd to 3rd Avenues between 32nd and 37th Streets; 718-965-6450, industrycity.com

4. **Li-Lac Chocolates** 68 35th St.; 212-924-2280, li-lacchocolates.com

5. **Industry City Distillery** 33 35th St.; 718-305-6951, drinkicd.com

6. **Bush Terminal Park** West of 1st Avenue and south of 43rd Street; nycgovparks.org

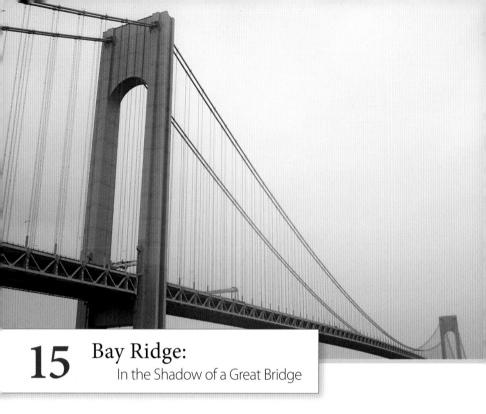

15 Bay Ridge:
In the Shadow of a Great Bridge

BOUNDARIES: Senator St., 4th Ave., John Paul Jones Park, Shore Pkwy.
DISTANCE: 5.2 miles
SUBWAY: R to Bay Ridge Ave. (68th St. exit)

Unlike many Brooklyn neighborhoods with "Hill" in their name, Bay Ridge actually sits on elevated ground—a bluff overlooking Upper New York Bay. It was the proximity to and views of the water that attracted Manhattan's elite in the late 1800s, when Bay Ridge developed as a summer resort. The extension of the subway system in 1915 opened the neighborhood to the middle class, and it became more urbanized. It may appear more suburban to you, as there are plenty of freestanding houses with lawns where this walk is focused—west of 3rd Avenue, away from the commercial corridors of 3rd, 4th, and 5th Avenues. The neighborhoods from Bay Ridge south to

Bensonhurst have long been identified with Italian Americans but more recently gained Russian, Middle Eastern, and Chinese populations. You can still find several Irish pubs in Bay Ridge, but the Norwegian food shops are gone. One constant: throughout the years this *has* remained one of the best places in Brooklyn to enjoy the water.

Walk Description

With the church to your right, walk one block north on 4th Avenue and make a left on Senator Street. Past the Gothic-style school on your right come the residences that earned this block a spot on the National Register of Historic Places. Bay Ridge is not one of Brooklyn's brownstone neighborhoods, but don't tell that to the lions on guard here at the top of every stoop. Brownstone was actually passé by the time construction of these homes began in 1906; bowfront Renaissance Revival row-houses like these tend to be limestone. Both sides of the street were developed by one company, and there *are* differences among the houses—look at the ornamentation around the windows.

Turn left on 3rd Avenue, then right on 68th Street. Bay Ridge has a number of one-block streets and even half-block streets with an outlet at only one end. A fine example is on your left: Madeline Court, a slate-roofed enclave demarcated with brick gateposts. Note that the garages on 68th Street architecturally match the houses.

Across Ridge Boulevard, find some of those aforementioned limestone bowfront rowhouses on your right, also with lion heads atop the banisters. Farther along, Bay Cliff Terrace on the left is another Tudor cul-de-sac. The row of bowfronts down here on your right are notable for their elegant doorways with colored-glass transoms.

At Colonial Road, you can detour into ❶ **Owl's Head Park.** The "EWB" in the shield on the fence was Eliphalet W. Bliss, a mogul whose mansion stood on this site; some longtime residents still call this Bliss Park. It has excellent views of One World Trade Center from its playground near 67th Street and of the harbor from the hill and paved terrace at its south end. Bliss purchased the estate from Henry C. Murphy, a founding editor of the *Brooklyn Eagle*. In his lifetime Murphy served as mayor of Brooklyn, ambassador, and congressman, but it's because of his act as state senator drafting the bill authorizing construction of the Brooklyn Bridge that Senator Street is named for him.

From alongside the park on 68th Street, turn left on Bliss Terrace.

Turn right on Bay Ridge Avenue, a formal street name generally forsaken by locals in favor of the numerical designation, 69th Street. Past all the brick on the left, two houses with porches from the first decade of the 20th century flank a couple of commercial buildings and give you an idea of what Bay Ridge looked like prior to its widespread development. Cross Narrows Avenue en route to Shore Road. Continue straight ahead onto the 600-foot-long American Veterans Memorial Pier, with an awesome panorama entailing the Verrazano-Narrows Bridge, the Statue of Liberty, and a unique vantage point on the Hudson River as it empties into Upper New York Bay. Gazing full-on at Manhattan's southern tip—the Hudson separating it from New Jersey, the East River branching off to the right—you can just imagine the view of the Twin Towers this pier used to offer. That's why Brooklyn's 9/11 memorial was placed here. It's shaped like a firefighter's trumpet, used in the 18th century, as sirens are today, to warn of a fire.

Go back to Shore Road and make a right. Opposite the condo at #6917, enter the ❷ **Narrows Botanical Gardens,** a wonderful 4.5-acre oasis created and maintained by volunteers (keep that in mind in case you can't access certain sections). First stop is the native plant garden on the right, which aims to re-create Brooklyn's landscape of 400 years ago, before European colonization, not to mention industrialization. Wandering south, you'll encounter gardens dedicated to cacti, roses, fragrant plants, and pollinators. Make your way to the alley of linden trees leading to the arched gate at 71st Street. Exiting onto Shore Road, go to your left and keep an eye out for the lily pond.

Go onto Mackay Place across from the lily pond. The small lot on your right at Narrows Avenue was the ❸ **Barkuloo family's burial ground** from 1725 to 1848, and Revolutionary War soldiers are among those interred here. You should be able to unlatch the gate and enter to read about some of the family history.

Proceed on Mackay Place, taking a peek down Louise Terrace to your left. Louise was a middle name of Mr. Mackay's wife; this society family was outraged when granddaughter Ellin married someone in showbiz—even though that someone was Irving Berlin.

Turn right on Colonial Road.

Turn left on 76th Street and ascend the staircase. The ridge at this point was too steep for vehicles, so steps were installed to accommodate pedestrians. The house on the right at the top of the stairs, with a front door and porte cochère seemingly borrowed from a medieval castle, was built in 1900 for the founder of Blue Cross. The mansion opposite, its circular columned portico facing the water, dates to 1865.

Turn right on Ridge Boulevard, within the approximately eight-by-three-block area where Bay Ridge's grandest homes are concentrated. On your left at 80th Street stands Union Church, founded when a Dutch Reformed congregation on the site merged with a Presbyterian church located a block away. It erected this building in 1924, retaining the original Reformed structure of 1896 for the front of the sanctuary.

Turn right on 82nd Street. This block has a sampling of early-20th-century homes, and also a sampling of how some of those homes have been altered or replaced with far less charming dwellings. (If you're willing to add on to an already long walk, go in the other direction on 82nd, then loop back to this point via 3rd Avenue and 81st Street, and you'll see more old homes, including turn-of-the-century Victorians.)

At Narrows Avenue, make a left. One fanciful house and its expansive lawn occupy the entire side of the block to your right. Resembling a cottage out of a fairy tale, it's been nicknamed the ❹ **Gingerbread House** but is officially the Howard E. and Jessie Jones House. While this 1917 construction presents the hominess and natural materials (those rocks!) that are hallmarks of the Arts and Crafts movement, the roof thatching is merely simulated.

Turn right on 83rd Street and walk alongside Fort Hamilton High School.

Turn right on Shore Road. Note the trilevel fountain on the grounds at 82nd Street. Go as far as 80th Street to see a few more sumptuous properties.

Across Shore Road, the flagstaff with yardarm honors the Spanish-American War victory and goes by the moniker Old Glory Lookout. Walk downhill via either path next to it, then onto the pedestrian bridge over the Belt Parkway—a spot, incidentally, that is the westernmost point of Long Island.

Head south—toward the Verrazano-Narrows Bridge—on the paved ❺ **biking and walking path** hugging the shoreline. John Travolta wooed his leading lady from one of these benches in *Saturday Night Fever,* whose hero lived (and boogied) in Bay Ridge.

Take the next pedestrian bridge back across the highway, coming through Shore Road Park. Go to the right back at Shore Road.

Turn left on 95th Street. On your left, the pale yellow house with green shutters and a lovely porch is the oldest house in Bay Ridge, built circa 1847.

Return to Shore Road and make a left to continue in the direction you'd been going. Check out Fontbonne Hall Academy at 99th Street. This Spanish Mission villa, the only 19th-century home still standing on Shore Road, was built as a summer estate and later purchased by corpulent railroad tycoon Diamond Jim Brady for his showgirl paramour Lillian Russell.

Go two more blocks on Shore Road, then cross 4th Avenue and head straight into ❻ **John Paul Jones Park,** aka Cannonball Park, for reasons you see to your left. Its obelisk commemorates the WWI naval heroics of the Dover Patrol. Look also for the boulder nearby paying tribute to the Battle of Brooklyn—which began when British troops came ashore at a wharf that today would be under the Verrazano Bridge. On the other side of the lawn, a low-lying monument recognizes the efforts of one John LaCorte to promote the achievements of Italian Americans; thanks to Signor LaCorte, the bridge above you is named not only for the water it traverses (the Narrows strait links Upper and Lower New York Bay) but also for the Italian who was the first European

Extend Your Bay Ridge Walk

From Cannonball Park, you can return to the waterside path and head to Bensonhurst or pay a visit to **Fort Hamilton** and its Harbor Defense Museum. Make a right on 101st Street and go one block to reach Fort Hamilton. One of the nation's oldest continuously garrisoned forts, it was constructed between 1825 and 1831 and is used primarily at present for recruitment and new-enlistee processing. At security, say you're here for the museum. You can see the houses of Colonels' Row and cannons from various eras across the road from the security center. The free-admission **Harbor Defense Museum,** located inside the caponier—a structure that protected the fort from a land assault—displays a collection of artifacts, uniforms, pictures, and models spanning more than two centuries of New York military history. Outside the museum, you are permitted to remain on the grounds within the original fort, as indicated by a granite-block wall (the newer section is still home to about 600 families, plus some federal offices). The landmarked Fort Hamilton Community Club was once the officers' club but today is a membership club for federal employees. On its south side is a bluff from which you have an expansive view of the water and can see down to Coney Island's Parachute Jump.

Want to walk some more along the bay? From outside Cannonball Park on 4th Avenue, cross Shore Road and the Belt Parkway on-ramp to get onto the sidewalk. Traverse the overpass, then head downhill to your left and back onto the waterside path. Walk under the bridge. Bypass the next pedestrian bridge over the parkway, about a mile along; it's another half mile to the second pedestrian bridge. Cross this one into Bath Beach Park. Follow the walkway through to 17th Avenue, go right on Bath Avenue, and then left on 18th Avenue into **Bensonhurst**—Brooklyn's Italian American stronghold (though now diversified). The elevated train at 86th Street is the one Gene Hackman chased in his car in *The French Connection;* John Travolta's opening strut of *Saturday Night Fever* also took place on 86th Street in Bensonhurst. Continue north on 18th Avenue to New Utrecht Reformed Church, on your right between 84th and 83rd Streets. New Utrecht was one of the five towns established by the Dutch in the 17th century in what would eventually become Brooklyn, and those early settlers founded the church, which has been on this site since 1699, in this building since 1828. Its flagpole was first erected in 1783 to celebrate victory in the American Revolution, thus earning the status of "liberty pole." Two blocks farther, across 82nd Street, is another Revolutionary War–related site, Milestone Park.

explorer to sail into New York Harbor. About 8,000 people, many of them Italian American, were displaced when the bridge was erected in 1964. Its 4,260 feet was the longest of any suspension bridge in the world at the time and is still the longest in the United States.

Leave the park at 4th Avenue and 101st Street. See the sidebar above for additional exploring from here, but if you're (understandably) ready to wrap up, go to the right on 4th Avenue. This area used to be nicknamed Irishtown, and Bay Ridge still has its own St. Patrick's Day parade, which steps off from St. Patrick's Church, on your right at 95th Street. The subway is just ahead on 4th Avenue.

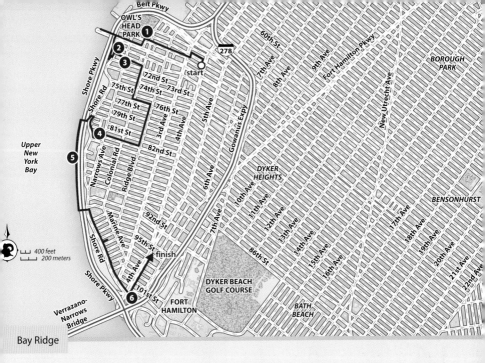

Points of Interest

1. **Owl's Head Park** 3rd Avenue and Colonial Road; nycgovparks.org

2. **Narrows Botanical Gardens** Shore Road between Bay Ridge Avenue and 72nd Street; narrowsbg.org

3. **Barkuloo Cemetery** Mackay Place and Narrows Avenue

4. **Gingerbread House** 8200 Narrows Ave.

5. **Belt Parkway shore path** West of Belt Parkway between 80th and 92nd Streets

6. **John Paul Jones Park** 4th Avenue and Shore Road; nycgovparks.org

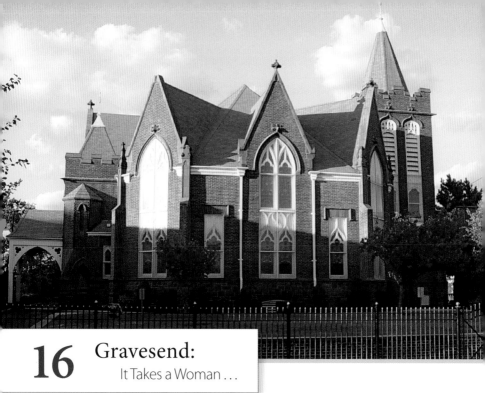

16 Gravesend:
It Takes a Woman ...

Above: Trinity Tabernacle on Neck Road

BOUNDARIES: Ave. P, Ocean Pkwy., Gravesend Neck Rd., Van Sicklen St.
DISTANCE: 3 miles
SUBWAY: F to Kings Hwy. (Ave. S exit)

One hundred and forty-four years before the United States adopted its Constitution, a town was founded on the ideals of religious, social, and political freedom and equal rights for all. It was the first of the six original settlements of Brooklyn, and the only non-Dutch one among them. Most extraordinary of all, its founder was a woman, Lady Deborah Moody. The baron's widow had left Massachusetts, her first home in the New World, because it was too restrictive—puritanical, one might say—on personal liberties. Gravesend, the town she established in 1643 and received a land patent for in 1645, started as 28 lots on 17 acres but eventually grew to encompass the entire southern sector of present-day Brooklyn (including Coney Island). This walk explores Lady

Moody's stomping grounds and illuminates how Gravesend's architectural and cultural character has changed over the years.

Walk Description

Come down from the train onto McDonald Avenue. Walking around Gravesend, you'll notice the presence of two ethnic groups in particular—Italians and Sephardic Jews (hailing primarily from the Middle East, especially Syria). Both have been in the area since the early 20th century, but while the number of Italian Americans here is dwindling, the Jewish population has been growing since the 1990s. It won't take long for you to spot signs of both communities: a large kosher supermarket is next to the train on the east side of McDonald. Walk south on McDonald, and after crossing Avenue S, you'll see bocce courts inside McDonald Playground on your left.

Enter McDonald Playground at the first gate, walk past the bocce courts, and on the other side of the comfort station look for the four square panels engraved with scenes of life in old Gravesend. Then return to McDonald Avenue and go left.

Use the first crosswalk you can to get to the other side of McDonald Avenue. Tucked between wings of the massive Magen David Yeshivah (a Sephardic school) is a compact white house at #2138. Known as ❶ **Hubbard House,** it was built circa 1830, with the taller wing added in the 1920s. The same woman (a daughter of Italian immigrants) lived here from 1904 until her death in 1997; the subsequent owner successfully campaigned for a landmark designation.

Turn right on Avenue T. The first house on the right, at the McDonald corner, is identifiable from its shape and roof as an early-20th-century frame house. There are still quite a few of them around Gravesend, but many have been even more severely altered, to the point that you can barely detect their age and original appearance. Before you even reach Lake Street, you'll likely espy the tall and somewhat unusual tower of Sts. Simon & Jude Church, which was established in 1897 but obviously not in this building. The real looker, though, is the church's former school across the street, where the ❷ **Coney Island Prep** charter high school opened in 2013. Check out the cornerstone on the right that says RELIGION SCIENCE PATRIOTISM (not something every Christian school would carve in stone), then look up from there to the eagle at the top corner.

Make a left on Van Sicklen Street. Across Avenue U on your left is another dramatic school building, this one erected in 1913 in the Collegiate Gothic style, complete with terra cotta parapet and gargoyles.

Turn left on Gravesend Neck Road, stepping within the bounds of the original town of Gravesend. Lady Moody was a visionary of urban planning as well as socio-politics. She laid out a rectangular grid of four quadrants, each with an equal number of lots and a commons at the center—a design regarded as a forerunner of modern urban planning. Gravesend Neck ran east–west through the middle of the grid, McDonald Avenue (then Gravesend Avenue) was the village's central north–south artery. The house at #27, on your left, sits on land that was partially in Lady Moody's own lot, but she never lived in the house, which was built in the 1700s or maybe the late 1600s, making it one of Brooklyn's oldest houses. Its owners from 1904 to 1913—who added the dormers—started calling it ❸ Lady Moody's House, and the label stuck even after its authenticity was debunked. Across the street are two cemeteries where Gravesend's original settlers and American Revolution soldiers were interred, though virtually all the 17th-century headstones have crumbled away or are illegible.

Turn left on McDonald Avenue, then left on Village Road North, the northern boundary in Lady Moody's town design. On your left, #38 is a Dutch Colonial from the mid-1800s, known as the ❹ Ryder–Van Cleef House. The house at #32 was built around 1788 as a school (which George Washington visited) and later used as Gravesend's town hall. Both buildings have been relocated from their original sites.

Cross Lake Street and go into Lady Moody Triangle. After looking at its granite monument memorializing World War II and the founding of Gravesend, cross Avenue U, a main commercial thoroughfare of southern Brooklyn and a good place for Italian food. Head to the right.

Continue east on Avenue U and you'll see more Italian names on shops and businesses. Turn right on West Street, and when it forks after a block, go to the right onto Village Road East—the eastern perimeter of Lady Moody's Gravesend.

Turn left at Gravesend Neck Road, often called simply Neck Road. Past West Street, the gospel church ❺ Trinity Tabernacle occupies a building constructed in 1893 as the third house of worship for a Dutch Reformed congregation founded in 1655. The Victorian parsonage next to the church dates to 1901.

Veer left at the traffic triangle, onto Avenue V, walk four residential blocks to ❻ Ocean Parkway, and turn left. Now that you've experienced Lady Moody's 17th-century masterstroke of urban planning, here's one from a couple of hundred years later. Ocean Parkway was created by Frederick Law Olmsted and Calvert Vaux in their Prospect Park design, one of two landscaped boulevards radiating from the park (Eastern Parkway is the other) and extending nature out into the city. Ocean Parkway stretches south from the park all the way to the Coney Island boardwalk. This section through Gravesend has become a primo location for Sephardic families' opulent homes. To your left, #2134 was put on the market in 2012 for $14 million—the most ever asked for a single-family home in Brooklyn. Its sidewalks are heated to melt the snow.

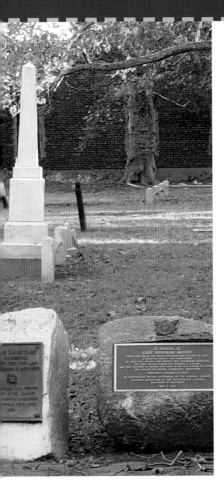

A plaque (right) in Gravesend's colonial-era cemetery commemorates town founder Lady Moody

On the next block, Congregation Shaare Zion is the Sephardics' flagship synagogue. The Gravesend area has the biggest Syrian Jewish population of anywhere in the United States, and it overlaps with the large Orthodox Jewish community centered in neighboring Midwood (east of Ocean Parkway).

Turn left at Avenue T, looping back to Ocean Parkway via right turns on East 3rd Street and Avenue S through pleasant suburban-style streets. Back at Ocean Parkway, go left. Walk at least a few blocks on the grassy median mall, where you can take a break on a bench. North of Avenue R, you'll cross Kings Highway, which once upon a time connected the original settlements of Kings County. It also was purportedly the first US road designated "highway." Ocean and Eastern, meanwhile, were the first two dubbed "parkway"— a word Olmsted invented.

At Avenue P, check out the Art Deco apartment building at #1601 on the right, but then turn left. To call the Venetian development, on your right at East 3rd Street, ambitious is obviously an understatement—a bit too ambitious, apparently, as its building costs came in at twice what had been estimated.

One block farther, you can catch the F train at McDonald Avenue.

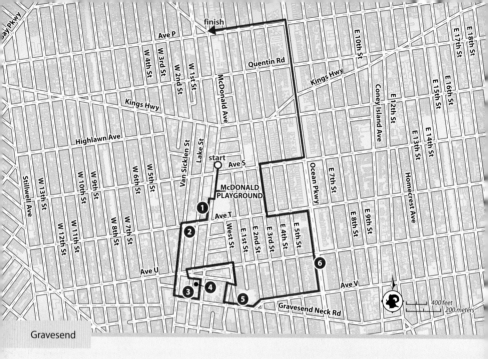

Gravesend

Points of Interest

1 Hubbard House 2138 McDonald Ave.

2 Coney Island Prep 294 Ave. T; 718-676-1063, coneyislandprep.org/our-schools/high-school

3 Lady Moody's House 27 Gravesend Neck Road

4 Ryder–Van Cleef House 38 Village Road N.

5 Trinity Tabernacle 121 Gravesend Neck Road; 718-998-7827, trinitytab.com

6 Ocean Parkway Avenue V to Avenue P

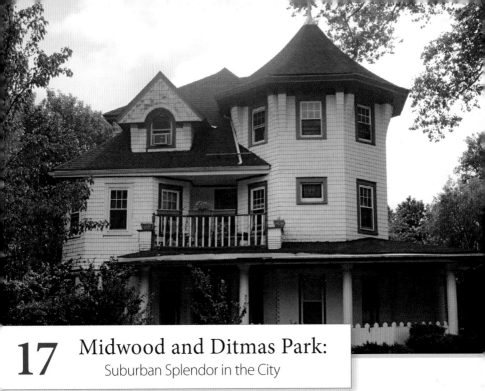

17 Midwood and Ditmas Park:
Suburban Splendor in the City

Above: *A home on Avenue H in Fiske Terrace*

BOUNDARIES: Dorchester Rd., Flatbush Ave., Ave. H, E. 16th St.
DISTANCE: 3 miles
SUBWAY: 2 or 5 to Flatbush Ave./Brooklyn College

In the 1650s, Dutch colonists established five towns in what would become Brooklyn. One of them was alternately called Midwout or Vlackebos—both names referred to woods, and both were eventually anglicized, to Midwood and Flatbush. Today these two neighborhoods account for a large swath of central Brooklyn directly south of Prospect Park, and they entail about a dozen mini-neighborhoods originally developed as suburban communities around the turn of the century. Some people, especially those who don't live here, do not bother with any distinctions: Flatbush is Flatbush, Midwood is Midwood, and what ya talkin' about with Nottingham, Caton Park, Homecrest, and so forth? This walk takes you through a few of

Midwood's sub-neighborhoods and from there into Ditmas Park, part of Victorian Flatbush—which is not strictly Victorian in style or age. This is a residential route that stays off of Midwood's major commercial streets.

Walk Description

From the busy intersection where you emerge from the subway, walk on Hillel Place to the ❶ **Brooklyn College** gate on Campus Road. This public university held its first classes in Downtown Brooklyn in the late 1920s and built this campus in 1937, with $5 million in New Deal funds. You enter at the school's newest addition, the Leonard & Claire Tow Center for the Performing Arts, made possible by a $10 million gift from the namesake alumni, who met as Brooklyn College students (and also endowed a theater at Lincoln Center). Just behind it is the Brooklyn Center for the Performing Arts, which books well-known artists and touring productions in the 2,400-seat Walt Whitman Theatre. But follow the path from the Tow Center leading farther onto the campus, passing Whitehead Hall on the right as you proceed to the college's emblematic structure, its Georgian-style library.

Walk alongside the front of this cupolaed clocktower (formally named La Guardia Hall), and at the other end, go left and you'll find the Lily Pond on your right. Roam here as much as you wish, then head back toward the library building and go down the stairs in front, taking note of the Martin Luther King Jr. bust. Alumni of this "poor man's Harvard" include novelist Irwin Shaw, film director Paul Mazursky, attorney Alan Dershowitz, US senator Barbara Boxer, author Frank McCourt, and actor Jimmy Smits.

Exit on the far side of the green, at Bedford Avenue. Across Bedford to your left, Roosevelt Hall (with cupola) was the school's original gym; President Franklin D. Roosevelt laid its cornerstone in 1936, proud to support an institution that would provide educational opportunities for the nonwealthy as well as employment during the Depression for construction workers.

Go to the right on Bedford Avenue. Pass under the enclosed bridge connecting older and newer sections of Midwood High School. Built by the WPA in 1940, the school was designed for 2,800 students but now has about 4,000. They can select a concentrated field of study, similar to a college major, and may take classes at Brooklyn College free of charge. Woody Allen went to school here, as did *Man v. Food* star Adam Richman, cartoonist Roz Chast, Blondie's Chris Stein, poet June Jordan, and indie filmmaker Noah Baumbach.

Turn left on Glenwood Road. This area is known as South Midwood, although it's actually north of Midwood proper (the "South" may have been a reference to Flatbush's boundaries). It was created after a real estate company named Germania purchased the farmland of John Lott in the 1890s. Germania created infrastructure, paved the streets, and set property covenants, but sold off lots to developers and individual buyers for actual home construction. Their advertisements pitched a clean, green community "away from the riff raff and rabble of the city."

Turn left on East 21st Street, or Kenmore Place in South Midwood's original layout.

Turn right at Campus Road, opposite Brooklyn College's athletic fields. That ❷ **Hot Spot Tot Lot** on your right isn't just a cutesy name—it's an homage to the college's heating plant, which you pass as you turn right onto Avenue H. It's one of the campus's original structures, erected in 1936.

Upon crossing Ocean Avenue, see the gatepost to the left, erected to mark entrée into Fiske Terrace, another suburb-in-the-city development from the same era as South Midwood. The majority of its houses were built between 1905 and 1907.

Make a right on East 18th Street to see one of the only pre-1900 homes—it's the fourth on the left after the corner house. Built in 1898, #808 still looks spiffy with its round porch, Palladian window, and wreath ornamentation. This house and the severely modified #790 (1899) are the only Fiske Terrace houses constructed on land owned by Mr. Fiske; the community was really developed by the T. B. Ackerson Company after it had purchased Fiske's land.

Return to Avenue H and continue in the direction you'd been going. On your left at East 16th Street, that's not a rural general store but a ❸ **subway station house.** It was constructed in 1906, as Ackerson's sales office, and is the only station house in the entire system that was converted from another use. It's also one of the few left made of wood.

Turn around and go back to East 17th Street and make a left to see more residences of Fiske Terrace—including those down Wellington or Waldorf Court. While houses were built according to a few basic models and certain elements recur, they generally look different from one another: developers had learned from the rowhouse construction of the late 1800s, which gave us those uniform—albeit highly prized today—brownstones.

Turn right on Glenwood Road. Among the rules for original property owners of Fiske Terrace was a minimum construction cost, and it was higher if you were building on Glenwood than on a numbered street.

Turn left on East 19th Street. Now you're in Midwood Park, which arose, like South Midwood, from Germania's acquisition of Lott farmland. It had a different developer than Fiske Terrace but has similar homes and covers the same streets, just north of Glenwood. At Foster Avenue are ❹ **brick gateposts** marking the northern border of Midwood Park.

Continue north, and when you reach Newkirk Avenue, you enter Ditmas Park, developed by a nonpracticing attorney named Lewis Pounds starting in 1902. It's a smorgasbord for the eyes; most houses could be described as freely interpreted Colonial Revival styles. This block includes three by Pounds's preferred architect, Arlington Isham—#535, 521, and that fantastic last one on the left (1904), which *really* takes advantage of its corner lot.

Turn left on Ditmas Avenue. Isham designed the two homes facing the avenue on the right, circa 1902.

Turn right on East 18th. There's much to admire all along the block, right down—er, up—to smaller details, like that face atop #488 and the storybook oriel on #472. That house and the one to the right of it came before Ditmas Park as a whole, their year of construction placed at 1899. On your right near the end of the block, the multisided bulge topped by a pyramidal roof with tall dormer windows belongs to the parish house of the ➎ Flatbush-Tompkins Congregational Church.

Turn right on Dorchester Road for a look at the church itself, but then head in the other direction.

Turn left on East 17th. Isham designed no fewer than 10 of the houses on this block, including the first three on the left. That loggia on #455 is sometimes called a sleeping porch, as it was a cool place to spend a summer night pre-air-conditioning. Within this bounty of classic Victoriana, #444, 471, and 484 are especially delightful.

Go right on Ditmas Avenue. In the 1910s, Mary Pickford and Douglas Fairbanks Jr., Hollywood's original power couple, lived on Ditmas two blocks west of here. The movie biz was still based on the East Coast then, and they were working at Vitagraph, a studio in Midwood. (Vitagraph was eventually folded into Warner Bros.; the studio, located at East 14th near Avenue M, was used by NBC into the 1980s.)

Turn left on East 16th. This entire block consists of Isham's 1909 adaptations of the California bungalow style—except for the last two on the right, #574 and 578, which were built in the 1880s and later transported to these lots.

Turn right on Newkirk Avenue, and the B/Q train is to your left—on the sunken "open cut," which residents preferred to underground or elevated when the city eliminated all street-level rail crossings.

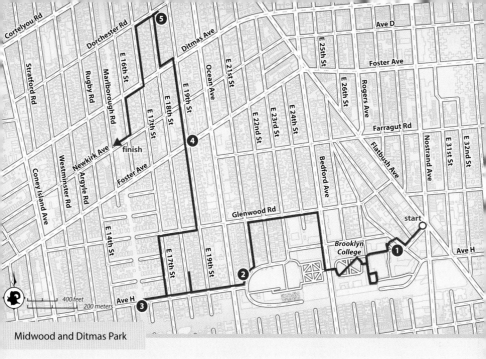

Midwood and Ditmas Park

Points of Interest

1. **Brooklyn College** 2900 Bedford Ave., 718-951-5000; brooklyn.cuny.edu
2. **Hot Spot Tot Lot** Campus Road and East 21st Street; nycgovparks.org
3. **Avenue H subway station** Avenue H and East 16th Street
4. **Midwood Park gateposts** Foster Avenue at East 17th, 18th, and 19th Streets
5. **Flatbush-Tompkins Congregational Church** 424 E. 19th St.; 718-282-5353

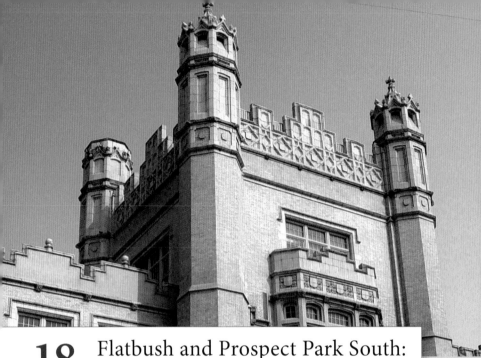

18 Flatbush and Prospect Park South: Town and Country

Above: *The central tower of Erasmus Hall High School*

BOUNDARIES: Church Ave., Bedford Ave., Cortelyou Rd., Westminster Rd.
DISTANCE: 3.9 miles
SUBWAY: B or Q to Church Ave. (Church Ave. exit)

Even before Brooklyn became familiar to everyone, Flatbush was one of its neighborhood names recognized by non–New Yorkers. They'd heard of Flatbush from the movies (it's in the title of several), from the Dodgers (who actually played in Crown Heights), and from local boys and girls made good (there are a lot of them!). Virtually all the black-and-white images and clichés about "growing up in Brooklyn" sprang from the streets of Flatbush, as did the writers, filmmakers, and sentimentalists who spread them around the world. At the turn of the century, developers created posh suburban-style communities in the area—with varied freestanding homes on spacious lots and plenty of grass and trees—that are now known collectively as Victorian Flatbush. The glorious homes here, not all of them strictly Victorian in style, are a hidden gem of residential Brooklyn.

Walk Description

Cross Church Avenue and walk south on East 18th Street, watching on the right for the unglamorous entrance to the ❶ **Knickerbocker Field Club** (est. 1889). Go in and check it out. In its more exclusive days, "The Knick" was primarily a place for socializing and dining, although it's always had tennis courts. Its clubhouse contained a ballroom and a bowling alley.

Return to the gate. Upon leaving the club grounds, walk straight ahead onto Tennis Court. The club was developed in conjunction with this street—except it wasn't just a street originally. It was the first suburban development in Flatbush, lined with majestic homes on 50-foot-wide lots. Tennis Court the community didn't last, with some fine apartment buildings replacing the houses in the 1920s and '30s. Spend a few minutes examining the fantastic entry of the Chateau Frontenac (1929) opposite East 19th. Among its embellishments, the shield with fleurs-de-lis was a coat of arms of the French monarchy; various characters, like the dragon, were emblems of individual French kings.

Turn onto East 19th Street, but look back for a full view of the Chateau Frontenac and its elaborate architecture, right up to the tippy-tops.

Make a left at Albemarle Road. Just past Ocean Avenue, you've got another lavish entryway on the Arista apartments to your left and griffin reliefs on the building to your right.

Turn left on East 21st Street. Two cul-de-sacs to your right, Albemarle Terrace and Kenmore Terrace, constitute a historic district. Albemarle is lined with Federal-style brick rowhouses with small front lawns; Kenmore is more modern in appearance, though it was developed just two years later, in 1918. The freestanding house with a porch at the 21st Street end of Kenmore was a church parsonage. It dates to 1853, but that age may not impress you once you see the church it serves. . . .

Turn right onto Church Avenue from East 21st, beside the churchyard. If any of these ancient gravestones are legible, you'll see the names of the founding families of Brooklyn. Make a right on Flatbush Avenue in front of the Flatbush Dutch Reformed Church. They began holding services on this site in 1654; this building, the church's third, was completed in 1796.

Across the avenue, the gargantuan neo-Gothic edifice of limestone and terra cotta was constructed, from 1904 to 1911, for Erasmus Hall High School. Its many celebrity alumni include Barbra Streisand and Neil Diamond (who were classmates), Barbara Stanwyck, Bobby Fischer, Beverly Sills, music exec Clive Davis and cartoonist Joseph Barbera (of Hanna-Barbera). Erasmus Hall was chartered as a public school in 1896 but originated as the private ❷ **Erasmus Hall Academy,** New York State's earliest secondary school. If you can see into the courtyard, you should espy the statue of Erasmus, 16th-century Dutch philosopher, and behind it a weathered white house with a porch—the original 1787 schoolhouse. If you can't see anything in the courtyard, at least look up within the archway for an Erasmus bas-relief—then step back and look higher up, near the tops of the wings flanking the main tower, for gargoyle faces. Then continue along Flatbush.

Turn left at Snyder Avenue. As an independent city, Flatbush built the quaint town hall on your left in 1875. Two decades later, Flatbush was annexed by the city of Brooklyn. Now look to your right, opposite the school playground, at the building that says EBINGER BAKING COMPANY. At its peak, Ebinger's had more than 65 bakeshops around the boroughs and Long Island. They went out of business in 1972 and took the recipe for their most famous product, the Brooklyn blackout cake—made with chocolate pudding and named for the wartime blackouts—with them. Many bakeries have since conjured their own versions of the cake.

Go back to Flatbush Avenue and make a left. The Jehovah's Witnesses hall on your left at Albemarle Road was a movie palace, open from 1921 to 1984 with a seating capacity of over 2,600. There were also two moviehouses on Church and one farther down Flatbush, with more than 6,000 seats combined, but proceed to the next block of Flatbush for the grandest of them all: the ❸ **Kings Theatre.** It was called the Loew's Kings then, and 3,600 people at a time could see a *pick-chuh* here. After the theater closed in 1977, the city bought it to prevent its demolition—and it stood here, vacant and decaying, for over 30 years. It reopened for concerts and stage shows in 2015 following a two-year, $95 million renovation. Loew's didn't classify this as a "Wonder Theater" simply because of that entertaining terra cotta facade; the interior is just as baroque, with pink marble stairs, walnut paneling, one-ton chandeliers, and more . . . and all these features have been restored.

Past the Kings, turn left on Duryea Place, and at East 22nd Street, go into the parking lot and walk straight across. Come out on Bedford Avenue and go right. Soon you'll be walking alongside an Art Deco landmark: the Sears store opened in 1932, with Eleanor Roosevelt—then the First Lady of New York State, but not yet the United States—in attendance. ❹ **Sears Roebuck,** which started as strictly mail-order, was still fairly new to retail business at the time. They targeted shoppers coming in cars rather than by public transit; hence, the tall corner tower to catch their eye.

Make a right on Beverley Road, continuing around the store and then across East 22nd. You have to make a right on Flatbush, then a quick left to proceed on Beverley. After crossing Ocean Avenue, look for the sculptures above the first-floor windows on the corner building on your right. Is this old man exhausted or perplexed? A scholar or an artist?

Turn left on East 19th Street. You've entered Beverley Square, developed in the mode set by Tennis Court. Beverley Square's developer, T. B. Ackerson, would then take the model farther south and develop Fiske Terrace (Walk 17). Gotta love that onion-domed bay window at #214 and the tiny attic oriel at #223, though both residences are impressive overall—as are many of their neighbors on this highly individualistic block.

Turn right on Cortelyou Road, then right on East 18th.

Make a left on Beverley. Or is it Beverly? Not even the authorities have made up their mind. The subway station on your left at 16th has the *e*, but the 2 and 5 station east of here spells it Beverly. And so did Dean Alvord, the developer of Prospect Park South, as you can observe from the brick gateposts on your right at Marlborough Road. Prospect Park South is the swankiest development in Victorian Flatbush: Alvord envisioned a garden enclave within the city, so some streets have landscaped medians. He replaced numbered streets with British names, and added a greater air of exclusivity with the ❺ gateposts along Beverley and Church Avenue.

Turn right at Marlborough. Alvord's two main watchwords for Prospect Park South houses—picturesque and varied—are reflected throughout the neighborhood, starting with the very first home here on the left, whose doorway alone is full of extraordinary detail. This is one of more than 40 houses in Prospect Park South by John Petit, Alvord's chief architect (and architect of the Hearst Building in San Francisco). Petit also designed #208, an Italian villa uncommon for the area. Opposite it, he went with another rare style for the neighborhood, French Gothic, with ample use of Tudor arches. Petit's responsible as well for the medieval-influenced delight at #184—which at one time was the home of intrepid reporter Nellie Bly, who lived here after she had traveled around the world in record time. At the end, #159 is Prospect Park South's earliest house, from 1899.

Turn right at Church Avenue, passing ❻ **Temple Beth Emeth** on your right. The "Little Jewel Box," as this 1913 synagogue has been nicknamed, has its original stained glass, a marble pulpit, and a bronze arc to hold the Torah.

Go right on Buckingham Road. Its diverse dwellings range from Tudor to farmhouse to some just a little too creative for easy categorization. The Petit-designed #115 was reportedly home to a Gillette (of razor fame). Petit also gave Prospect Park South what became its most famous mansion, the pagoda-ish #131, known as the "Japanese House." Orientalism was in vogue among the upper class of the late 19th century, but usually just one room in a house was decorated in the style. Next to it, #143 has its own charming quirks, most noticeably the open-air tower.

Turn right on Albemarle Road. Check out the carved porch columns on the house to your right, as well as the busts (facing Buckingham) at the second-floor brackets. This house, the one next to it on Albemarle, and the one across the street are the oldest homes on Albemarle, built 1899–1902. That woodsy lot on the south side of Albemarle is where Dean Alvord's own home was located; it burned down, but some of its steps should be visible to the right inside the gate.

The Albemarle mansions date mostly from 1903 to 1907. Many were built for corporate big-wigs of the day. Elmer Sperry, founder of the gyroscope company Sperry-Rand (progenitor of Unisys), lived in the fanciful mansion on your right as you reach Marlborough. The house diagonally across from it was purchased in 2015 by actress Michelle Williams, who's given it a much-needed renovation. Next to it is another looker, despite the stucco refacing.

Make a right on Rugby Road. To your right, #101 was painted pink when it was used for the exterior of the boardinghouse where Meryl Streep's character lived in *Sophie's Choice*. Opposite it is a pseudo–Swiss chalet, and next to that a Spanish Mission abode—both by John Petit. A stained-glass oval is a nice detail of the last house on the right.

Turn left on Church, then left on Argyle Road. Another stained-glass panel graces the third house on the left, which was originally wood-shingled. The house next to it is highlighted by red brackets and arched windows. After that, quarter-moon windows and an eyebrow dormer provide your first sampling of the corner mansion's flamboyance—go left on Albemarle to take it all in. The home's 22 rooms include a ballroom with wet bar behind those cute windows up top. Back in 1990, this mansion portrayed Claus Von Bülow's Newport estate in *Reversal of Fortune*. Across Albemarle from it is a Petit beauty with a true wraparound porch—go a few steps down Argyle to see all of the house.

With that block of Argyle to your left, head west on Albemarle. On your right, #1215 was designed in 1916 by William Van Alen and Craig Severance during their brief partnership. They would later be friendly rivals in a competition to build the world's tallest skyscraper. (Severance thought he'd won when his 927-foot Bank of Manhattan opened at 40 Wall Street in April 1930, but a month later it was surpassed by the Chrysler Building—Van Alen had secretly added a 125-foot spire to make it higher than Severance's building.) Next door on the left, a charmer by Petit has the initial *M* inscribed beneath the bay windows on the Westminster Road side, for May, surname of the first owner.

Cross Albemarle and walk south on Westminster. The double-balconied #126, built in 1902, was special enough that a renowned architect who *didn't* design it chose to live here: it was the home from 1907 to 1920 of Frank Helmle, who designed Prospect Park's beautiful Boathouse and Tennis House, plus several auspicious Brooklyn banks and churches. The threesome of #171, 173, and 177 offers a bounty of enchanting details, and the latter two date to pre-1900.

Turn left on Beverley Road. To your left are the only two Prospect Park South houses that face Beverley (on your right would be Beverley Square). Now make a right on Argyle. Halfway down the block, twin Victorians with conical turrets face each other . . . well, they probably were twins before painting and other alterations. At the end on your right, the last remaining cast-iron street sign from the early days of the area's development stands just inside the white picket fence.

Turn left on Cortelyou Road. The sidewalk clock at Rugby Road was installed along with the old-fashioned street lamps and Belgian-block sidewalk paving in a street upgrade circa 2006–07. Since then, several restaurants and boutiques have opened on Cortelyou. The Q subway is one block farther, just past Marlborough.

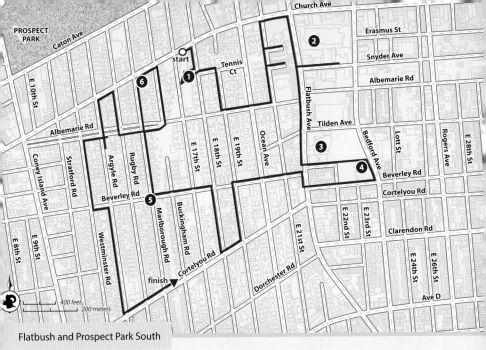

Flatbush and Prospect Park South

Points of Interest

1. **Knickerbocker Field Club** 114 E. 18th St.; 718-856-5098, knickerbockerfieldclub.net
2. **Erasmus Hall Academy** 911 Flatbush Ave.; 718-282-7804
3. **Kings Theatre** 1027 Flatbush Ave.; 718-856-2220, kingstheatre.com
4. **Sears Roebuck and Company store** Bedford Avenue and Beverley Road; 718-826-5800
5. **Prospect Park South gateposts** Beverley Road at Marlborough, Rugby, Argyle, Westminster, and Stratford Roads
6. **Temple Beth Emeth** 83 Marlborough Road; 718-282-1596, bethemeth.net

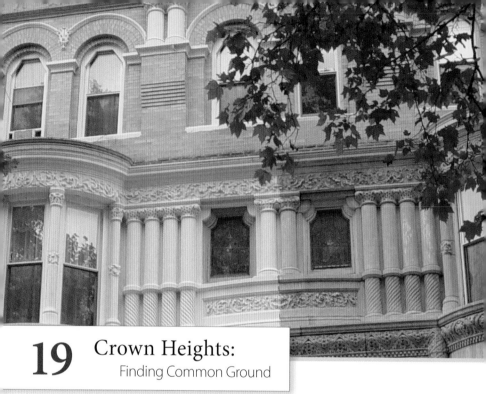

19 Crown Heights:
Finding Common Ground

Above: *Residential facades on St. Mark's Avenue*

BOUNDARIES: Pacific St., Albany Ave., President St., Franklin Ave.
DISTANCE: 4.1 miles
SUBWAY: 2, 3, or 4 to Kingston Ave.

"It seems to be not relevant for people who live here anymore," a homebuyer recently told *The New York Times* in reference to the 1991 Crown Heights riots. The riots—which shook up race relations, mayoral politics, and policing in the city—were touched off when a 7-year-old black child was fatally struck by a car in the motorcade of Rabbi Menachem Schneerson; a rabbinical student was stabbed to death by black men in retaliation during the three days of mayhem that ensued. So it's good that this ugly incident is no longer people's foremost association with Crown Heights, a neighborhood abounding with impressive old townhouses, mansions, and churches. Or is her comment proof that gentrifiers are divorced from their new community's history and the concerns and experiences of longstanding residents? (The white population north of Eastern Parkway has surged since 2005.) Regardless, Crown Heights has too long a history to be identified with only one event, and it has an ethnic heritage to be proud of: home to the most diverse West Indian population outside of the islands as well as to Hasidic Jews of the Chabad-Lubavitch sect.

Walk Description

On the south side of Eastern Parkway, Kingston Avenue is flanked by the Lubavitch world headquarters and the ❶ **Jewish Children's Museum.** A giant dreidel stands in front of the museum, where children of all faiths (and ages) are invited to learn about Jewish customs and history. They can, for example, "shop" and "cook" in a kosher store and kitchen, walk through a re-created shtetl, reenact biblical events with props, and play miniature golf on a course that takes them through the important events in a Jewish person's life.

Across Kingston is a block of Lubavitch buildings, but it's the one at #770 with three peaked gables that was the home of the Grand Rebbe who brought the movement to the United States in 1940, and as such it became central headquarters. Chabad centers around the globe are replicas of this building. Facilities within the Lubavitch complex include a synagogue, a school (yeshiva), a library, and a *kolel,* a Talmudic institute for married men.

Walk south on Kingston Avenue, the main commercial street of the Lubavitch community—grab a treat at the bakery if you're tempted by something in the window.

Turn right on President Street and enjoy two blocks of elegant to extravagant homes, built mostly during the first three decades of the 20th century.

Turn right on New York Avenue. Note the diamond-pane windows on the second house on the left. All the houses in this row originally had them—in fact, the houses were similar overall when constructed in 1909. They were marketed as single-family "American basement homes," which was a way of drawing attention to the absence of stoops (so they didn't actually have basements). Refacing and other alterations have made them a varied bunch.

Continue on New York Avenue across Eastern Parkway. This boulevard with landscaped pedestrian malls extends more than 3 miles from Prospect Park, and was created by park designer Frederick Law Olmsted to make nature an integral and continuous presence in the city. North of Eastern Parkway, the two blocks of New York Avenue on your left to St. John's Place were built by one developer in 1899. Those with swoop-shaped pediments on their doorways or dormer windows are faves.

Make a right on St. John's Place. At the end of the block, ❷ **St. Gregory's Catholic Church** was designed by Frank Helmle, architect of such Brooklyn landmarks as the Prospect Park Boathouse and the Williamsburgh Trust Company. This 1915 interpretation of an ancient Roman basilica has a terra cotta angel frieze.

Turn left on Brooklyn Avenue, or Carlos Lezama Way, per the street sign. In 1969, Mr. Lezama applied for a permit to hold a Carnival celebration along Eastern Parkway that in previous years had been confined to a block party. It grew into not only an annual event but one of the city's biggest: the West Indian American Day Parade, held on Labor Day and now attracting more than a million revelers every year.

Go left on Park Place. The first house on your right, with its fish-scale shingles and porch roof, provides a charming introduction to George Chappell, architect of many fine residences in the neighborhood. And it makes a picturesque Queen Anne pair with the larger house next to it that was built 13 years later, in 1899. Over on your left, a Victorian fortress extends down the second half of the block. It certainly seems too grand to be called a poorhouse, though it was constructed for that purpose by a Methodist church in 1889.

Make a right at New York Avenue, but go only as far as #190, home in the early 1950s to Ethel Waters, the famous blues singer and Oscar-nominated actress. On a 1954 episode of his TV show *Person to Person,* Edward R. Murrow interviewed Waters in her second-floor apartment. To the left of it, #196 is an 1891 work of George Chappell. Head back toward Park Place and turn right. You're greeted on the right by yet another Chappell design. This house gets a lot of its charm from its main entry, with portico and arched doorway, yet it has a second entrance to the left, with triangular pediment and Corinthian columns. On your left, the richly ornamented rowhouses came from another premier architect in Crown Heights, Axel Hedman.

Turn right on Nostrand Avenue, then right on Prospect Place. Hedman is responsible for the first row on your right (1901) and the five nonconsecutive brick houses on the left with central bay windows and vertical limestone "stripes" (1907). But the true delights on this block are the freestanding houses at #834, 836, and 847. Chappell seems to have had fun crowning his houses on this block: his work here includes #853 with orb-capped pointy roof, the exuberant duo across from it with urns atop stepped gables, and the two houses to their right whose gables culminate in roundish sculptings.

At New York Avenue, take a look at the double house facing you on the right—designed by Chappell in 1883—as well as its Prospect Place side once you've crossed the avenue. Farther down on the left, a set of slate-roofed white stucco cottages look charmingly misplaced. They were built in the early '20s and have garages behind them. Note that they share chimneys. A 1906 apartment house with fish and lions among its exquisite decor concludes the block.

Proceed into Brower Park and make your way to the other side. Then cross Kingston Avenue and continue on Prospect Place. Two sections of the block have been converted to plazas, outfitted with circular planters-cum-benches. These upgrades, including the sidewalk paving and globular streetlights, were created by architect I. M. Pei in the 1960s under hire by the community advocacy agency Bedford Stuyvesant Restoration Corporation—an implementation of ideas espoused by urban-renewal activist Jane Jacobs for open, well-lit, and pedestrian-friendly city streets.

Turn left on Albany Avenue, then left on St. Mark's Avenue, the other Pei "model block." Here, through traffic and curbside parking were eliminated altogether, trees were planted, and a playground installed. These redesigns aimed to allow for children's play and neighborly communing *and* to discourage drug dealers from hanging out. Among the honored guests at the unveiling of these two blocks in November 1969 was Ethel Kennedy, whose late husband, Robert F. Kennedy, had cofounded Bedford Stuyvesant Restoration as a US Senator representing New York.

Recross Kingston Avenue. The twin houses on the corner, which mirror each other and share a portico, ease you into the grandeur of the next two blocks. So prestigious was this address at the turn of the century, the whole area was called St. Mark's—and immediately recognized as a status symbol. How about that Beaux Arts mini-palazzo just before the church?

On the other side of the church is a nonmatching double house dating to 1891, followed by a mid-1890s pair amply adorned with colonettes. Then keep your eye out for the loggias on some houses a few doors down, including one shared by #855 and 857. This Romanesque stunner with corner cupola is an 1892 work by Montrose Morris, architect of several auspicious residences throughout brownstone Brooklyn. The twin-peaked houses next to it came courtesy of George Chappell in 1888. The imposing villa at the corner, built in 1870 for lumber magnate Dean Sage, was designed in 1870 by 33-year-old Russell Sturgis, who would gain greater renown as an art and architecture critic than practitioner.

To your left on Brooklyn Avenue is the entrance to the ❸ **Brooklyn Children's Museum,** founded in a mansion on this site in 1899. The first museum in the world with exhibits on a child-size scale tailored to child interests, it created the "hands-on" concept now used to engage visitors at countless museums. Inside this 1977 building—which has undergone a $43 million expansion—are a mini-zoo, a greenhouse, a block lab, and a play-learn area focused on places and cultures of Brooklyn, plus other exhibits.

With the museum on your right, head north on Brooklyn Avenue. Be sure to see the pointed tower with arched windows on this side of the Sage mansion. Cross Bergen Street to see the corner mansion on your left—a playful-looking Queen Anne thanks to its dormer windows of three different widths and the moldings around them that flare out at the bottom.

Turn your back to that house and walk east on Bergen Street. Continue past Kingston Avenue. Make a left on Revere Place, an enclave developed in its entirety in 1897. Anywhere you stand on the street, look to your left and to your right—the houses on both sides will be the same models. Also try to find the windows that still have stained-glass transoms.

Turn left on Dean Street. Back across Kingston, the first two houses on the left, radically altered though they may be, can still be recognized as golden oldies from their doors and roofs. When the homes were built in the 1870s, those mansard roofs were shingled, and the second floors had wooden shutters and no decks on top of the porches. Pass an apartment building and next on your left are Crown Heights' first brownstone rowhouses, dating to 1876. But even older is the ❹ Elkins House a little farther down on your right. Sitting on a generous elevated lot, this is the oldest residence in the whole neighborhood and the only freestanding wood home left from its era, built sometime between 1855 and 1869. It fell into extreme disrepair because it was looted after being left unlocked when vacated and was left to deteriorate for decades, but a recent buyer has filed plans for condos.

After the Elkins House, all the attached homes before the gap near the block's end are by George Chappell, 1892. Cross Brooklyn Avenue to the ❺ Queen Anne showplace constructed in 1887 for businessman-philanthropist John Truslow. Designed by the Parfitt Brothers, preeminent architects of the time, as a 50-room mansion, it eventually was subdivided into apartments and suffered decades of neglect, even while it was occupied. But it's looking splendid once again following a restoration by the affordable-housing developer that bought it in 2013. Tenants of the new apartments won the lottery, figuratively and literally: people with eligible incomes enter lotteries to be placed in subsidized apartments, but they rarely end up in a building that looks like this.

At the next corner, you probably need only take a few steps to the left for a good view of the Hebron Seventh Day Adventist Church across New York Avenue. This intriguing geometry primer features an octagonal sanctuary pierced with triangular gables above long arched windows. Built in the Byzantine Revival style for the First Church of Christ, Scientist, in 1909, it now serves a congregation of Haitian descent.

Cross New York Avenue and turn around to look at the church facing Hebron, the Union United Methodist Church, a powerful Romanesque presence of red brick and sandstone from 1891. Then continue west on Dean Street. On your left starting with #1228 is the neighborhood's second-oldest brownstone row, from 1877.

Cross Nostrand Avenue and find an amusing 1889 set by George Chappell on your left, beginning with the house with a stepped gable, followed by three clay-tile-roofed houses where the second-floor bay windows appear to be wearing skirts of shingles, then a home with an onion dome. And then the models repeat in reverse order! And just in case you haven't seen enough Chappell, enjoy the two rows that finish out the block on the left, starting with #1150. He's also responsible for the last six houses on the right.

Turn right on Bedford Avenue. The narrow building in the middle of the block, #1341, is a Chappell apartment house from 1888. And then you reach Montrose Morris's château-esque Imperial. When it was constructed in 1892, apartment living was uncommon for the well-to-do; to encourage them to try it, the building had to be opulent and the units spacious. It still looks swell on the outside; inside, apartment size has been shrunk by subdividing units.

Dip down Pacific Street to your right for a look at St. Bartholomew's, a late-19th-century country church, designed by Chappell. Turn to go back to Bedford Avenue, but on the way spend some time with the Bedfordshire, to your left at #1200, an apartment house Morris designed a year before the Imperial.

Back at Bedford, you can focus on the immense redbrick castle you'd no doubt already noticed: an armory built around 1892 for the National Guard's 23rd Regiment and used more recently as a homeless shelter. The regiment's World War I losses are paid tribute in a bronze tableau on the facade near Atlantic Avenue.

With the armory to your right, head down Bedford, staying to your left past the Imperial so you go onto Rogers Avenue. On your left across Dean, a senior center occupies the Union League clubhouse, erected in 1889. Look for the small busts of Abraham Lincoln and Ulysses S. Grant between the arches and the eagle with wings spread beneath the bay window on the right. The Union League, a Republican club, donated the statue across the street of General Grant astride his horse. The buildings on this part of Bedford also have ❻ **Grant Square** addresses.

Cross Rogers Avenue in front of Grant, then go left on the plaza behind him. You want to get a good look at the Washington Temple building on the next corner of Bedford Avenue, with faces in the column capitals. Built as a vaudeville house, it was a Loew's movie palace from the 1920s to the early '50s, when it closed and was taken over by what's now a Pentecostal megachurch. It was here that Reverend Al Sharpton preached his first sermon in 1959—at age 4.

Continue down Bedford, Brooklyn's "Automobile Row" in the 1920s. One of the last surviving showrooms is on your left at Sterling Place, and it still bears the name Studebaker, an automobile manufacturer that ceased production in 1966. This landmarked 1920 terra cotta building is now residential. Across Bedford, the New Life Tabernacle's building was originally a car showroom, but generations of New Yorkers knew it as Loehmann's. Frieda Loehmann opened the women's clothing store in 1921 and was here every day, dressed in black, patrolling from the second-floor landing. She's responsible for those dragons along the roofline (there are a couple on the roof

Weeksville Heritage Center

Weeksville Heritage Center, which can be added on to your Crown Heights or Bedford-Stuyvesant walk or visited separately, is built around the remnants of a 19th-century black community. A longshoreman named James Weeks established Weeksville in 1838, after slavery had been abolished in New York State. The oft-repeated description of it as a settlement of freed blacks is not entirely accurate: not all the people who lived there had been slaves, and quite a few were professionals, including teachers, ministers, the first black woman doctor in New York State (Susan McKinney Stewart), and the first black Brooklyn police officer (Moses Cobb).

Weeksville thrived for nearly a century, with about 300 residents at its peak, and included a nursing home, an orphanage, and a school (located where P.S. 243, aka the Weeksville School, now stands at Dean Street and Troy Avenue). At least three local churches that are still active—Bethel Tabernacle A.M.E., Berean Baptist, and St. Philip's—originated within Weeksville.

At the Heritage Center, you can tour the three extant Weeksville homes, which have been restored and furnished according to three different time periods to enlighten visitors about African American family life and historical events in 1860, 1900, and 1930. They are known as the Hunterfly Road Houses, after the country road on which they were built. Previously a Native American trail, Hunterfly disappeared in the 1910s when Brooklyn adopted a street grid—and the houses themselves virtually disappeared in the years that followed. They were discovered amid overgrowth behind Bergen Street rowhouses (since demolished) by a history teacher surveying the area from an airplane in 1968.

Weeksville Heritage Center (718-756-5250, weeksvillesociety.org) is at 158 Buffalo Ave., off St. Mark's Avenue. That's about two-thirds of a mile from the starting point of the Bed-Stuy walk or three-quarters of a mile from the midpoint (St. Mark's and Albany Avenue) of the Crown Heights walk.

too). In Loehmann's day, they were gilded—as was much of the interior. Though the store specialized in cut-rate designer clothes, it didn't look cheap inside; it was bedecked with stained glass, chandeliers, marble statues, and more. This Loehmann's store closed two months after Frieda's death in 1962.

Turn right on St. John's Place, then use a short street, St. Francis Place, to reach Lincoln Place and go right.

Wrap up at Franklin Avenue. The subway station is one block to the left, at Eastern Parkway. It's roughly a quarter mile west on Eastern Parkway to the Brooklyn Museum (see page 63). Or you can make a right from Lincoln onto Franklin and explore this newly trendy shopping and dining avenue. Opened on Franklin in the past five or so years is a slew of acclaimed restaurants plus cocktail bars, coffeehouses, specialty and vintage clothing boutiques, even a bookstore.

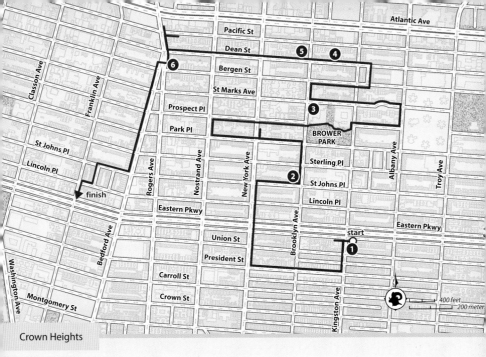

Crown Heights

Points of Interest

1. **Jewish Children's Museum** 792 Eastern Parkway; 718-467-0600, jcm.museum
2. **St. Gregory's Catholic Church** 224 Brooklyn Ave.; 718-773-0100, faithcommstgreg.org
3. **Brooklyn Children's Museum** 145 Brooklyn Ave.; 718-735-4400, brooklynkids.org
4. **Elkins House** 1375 Dean St.
5. **John Truslow House** 96 Brooklyn Ave.
6. **Grant Square** Bedford Avenue and Dean Street

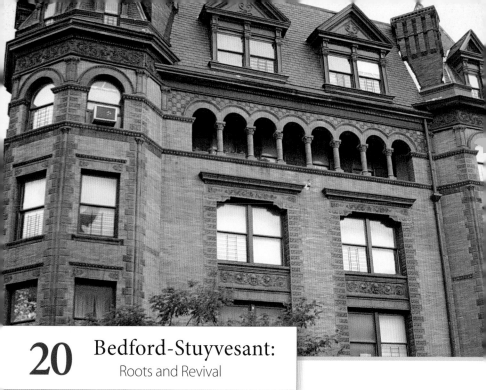

20 Bedford-Stuyvesant:
Roots and Revival

Above: The Alhambra apartment building occupies a full block of Nostrand Avenue between Macon and Halsey Streets

BOUNDARIES: Madison St., Stuyvesant Ave., Fulton St., Nostrand Ave.
DISTANCE: 3.1 miles
SUBWAY: A or C to Utica Ave.

"Bed-Stuy: Do or Die" is the mantra that emerged during the neighborhood's tough times of the '70s and '80s, an era captured in Spike Lee's movie *Do the Right Thing* and recaptured in Chris Rock's nostalgic sitcom *Everybody Hates Chris*. It was also during this time that Shawn Carter, later to be known as Jay-Z, was growing up in the Marcy Houses (located north of this route). Lately, however, some have modified the motto to "Do or Dine"—a reference to the burgeoning restaurant scene of this newly fashionable neighborhood. Gentrification has sent real estate prices soaring and left some concerned about its threat to their hometown's historic character. This walk begins in Stuyvesant Heights, a prosperous community of the late 19th century that eventually merged with Bedford, which had grown from a colonial-era farming village into a town.

Note: *You may wish to visit Weeksville at the start of this walk. See the sidebar on page 120.*

Walk Description

From the subway, walk west on Fulton Street. The school on your left isn't special to look at, aside from its Afrocentric murals, and has the generic name Boys and Girls High—but remember it; it will mean more later on the walk. Cross Stuyvesant Avenue and enter Fulton Park. Pass the pavilion and in-ground compass starburst, and walk through the bench-lined allée to the statue of steamboat inventor Robert Fulton. This is a bronze replica of a statue erected on the waterfront in 1872 (that's a model of the first Brooklyn steam ferry, *Nassau,* on Fulton's right).

Use the park exit to Fulton's right, and make a right on Chauncey Street.

Turn left on Stuyvesant Avenue. You really can't go wrong with any property on this block, but the faces between first-floor windows of the brownstones on your right and the extravagant doorways of the last limestone homes on your left are particularly delightful.

Make a left on Bainbridge Street. This attractive block has an entertaining assortment of designs on your right, multicultural faces sculpted into house facades on the left. Don't miss the children's faces above the doors of the third and fourth houses from the end on your right.

Make a right on Lewis Avenue. Across Decatur Street, the Southern restaurant Peaches—one of Bed-Stuy's popular new eateries—occupies the ground floor of the oldest apartment building in the neighborhood, dating to 1888.

Turn right on MacDonough Street. The Gothic church on your right with gargoyles perched from the tallest pinnacle was constructed in 1899 and since 1944 has been home to St. Philip's Episcopal, a congregation that sponsored the first black Boy Scout troop in the country.

Past the church, the mansions on both sides of the street were all built within a few years of one another, around 1870, and are among the oldest freestanding houses in the neighborhood. ❶ **Akwaaba,** the B&B at #347, was opened by a former editor-in-chief of *Essence* magazine and her husband in 1995—well before Brooklyn's tourism and hotel boom. It's been so successful they've added Akwaaba properties on the Jersey Shore and in Washington, DC, and the Poconos.

Turn left on Stuyvesant Avenue and walk four blocks included in a recent extension of the Stuyvesant Heights Historic District (first designated in 1971). On your right at Jefferson, ❷ **Bridge Street AME Church** is the oldest black congregation in Brooklyn, named for the street in Downtown where it was founded in 1818. It's been here since 1938 and has sponsored housing renovation and construction, a credit union, apartment buildings, and a senior center in the neighborhood.

Make a left on Jefferson Avenue. After crossing Lewis, you time-travel from the Victorian age to the Middle Ages. All that's missing is a moat around the castle (maybe that would keep it graffiti-free). Walk alongside it, then turn right on Marcus Garvey Boulevard to see the former 13th Regiment Armory from the front. As with several other colossal National Guard armories built in the late 1800s, construction of this one incited allegations of patronage and pork barreling. Its $700,000 final cost was more than twice what had been allotted, and the watchtower had to be reduced in height. The 13th Regiment was deactivated in 1971, and its armory is now a homeless shelter.

Head down Marcus Garvey Boulevard with the armory on your left. Cross Hancock Street, and before you cross the next street, look at the Halsey side of the duotone corner apartment building at #404. On the boulevard, you can see that it is one of four similar buildings, all designed in 1896. The next couple of blocks feature new bistros and signifiers of gentrification like a yoga studio, vintage boutique, and Citibike station amid bodegas and other old-school businesses.

Turn right on Decatur Street. Look down Albany Avenue on your left at the adjoining pair of houses at #1 and #3 and the apartment buildings on the other side of the street. There's a whole mix of styles and materials in the homes on this block of Decatur, including a quartet toward the end on the left with a checkerboard pattern on its taller end buildings. This group was constructed in 1889 as apartment buildings and, except for the fire escape, the two halves mirror each other. Farther along is the elegant Clermont apartment house at #79–81, designed in the 1890s by Montrose Morris—an eminent name in Bed-Stuy architecture, as you'll discover.

Go one more block on Decatur and make a left on Tompkins Avenue, followed by a quick right onto Fulton Street. Restoration Plaza, the retail and office complex on your left after Brooklyn Avenue, opened in the 1970s as a signature project of the Bedford Stuyvesant Restoration Corporation, the oldest community development corporation in the country. Restoration, as the agency is known, was founded in 1967 to spearhead local housing, cultural, educational, and economic development initiatives. Among them are the ❸ **Billie Holiday Theatre,** which produces new works by black playwrights, and the Center for Arts & Culture's Skylight Gallery (find out if an exhibition's on). Don't miss two exterior features of Restoration Plaza: first, the cows on the building facade—this used to be a milk-bottling plant—and second, the murals in the plaza up the steps opposite Marcy Avenue. They depict Restoration's founders, including Robert F. Kennedy (then a US Senator representing New York), and such African American icons as President Barack Obama and Bed-Stuy native Shirley Chisholm, the first black woman elected to the United States Congress (who made her own run for president in 1972).

Turn right on Marcy and walk through another plaza created (in 2013) by Restoration. Marcy Plaza's seating and landscaping occupy what previously had been part of the roadbed. The patterns within the colorful sidewalk mosaic at the MacDonough Street corner represent snippets of architecture from around the neighborhood. For example, the green diamonds close to the outer rim feature a pattern from a Fulton Park lamppost, while the black and white tiling that points into some of those green diamonds is modeled after the armory entrance. Most of the places depicted in this mosaic will be seen later on this walk—in the Bedford portion of Bedford-Stuyvesant.

Proceed three blocks and turn right on Hancock Street. Starting with the Queen Anne enchantress on the right corner, this block is filled with the work of Montrose Morris, a local resident who became one of Brooklyn's most influential residential architects. He designed the row at #236–244 in 1886 (the year he turned 25) essentially as model houses, showing prospective clients what he was capable of. The extravagantly ornamented brownstone-limestone #237 is not by Morris, but he was also responsible for #246–252 and #255–259, as well as the freestanding brownstone at #247, which many consider the belle of the block. Its owner of 30 years put it on the market in 2014 for $6 million, a top price tag in Bed-Stuy.

Make a left on Tompkins, an avenue where no fewer than eight new upscale apartment buildings are planned. Turn left on Madison Street and left on Marcy, coming around ❹ **Concord Baptist.** It's one of the country's largest black churches, with 12,000 members, an excellent choir, 160 years of history, and an active role in local political and social issues. Across the avenue stands the former Boys High School, a magnificent Romanesque structure built in 1891, with towers, dormers, and arches galore. Isaac Asimov, Norman Mailer, and Aaron Copland are among those who graduated from Boys High. Go another block on Marcy, and without turning, you should see the end pair of houses facing you on Jefferson. Their eye-catching features include cloche-capped carved posts at the stoops, above-door balconies, and stained-glass window panels.

Make a right on Jefferson, in front of Siloam Presbyterian Church, founded by an ex-slave in 1849. Siloam participated in the Underground Railroad (at an earlier location) and many subsequent civil rights battles. Malcolm X visited the church in 1964.

Turn left on Nostrand Avenue. On your right past Hancock is the ❺ⓐ **Renaissance,** Montrose Morris's 1892 masterstroke in brick and terra cotta. The next block has the even more sumptuous ❺ⓑ **Alhambra,** Morris's first major commission. It contained 30 nine-room apartments when it opened in 1889. Be sure to see the building from all three sides, on Halsey, Nostrand, and Macon.

To your left on Nostrand is another fabulous structure, Girls High School. The oldest public secondary-school building in New York City, it opened in 1886 and is the alma mater of Shirley Chisholm and Lena Horne. In the 1970s, it was merged with its male counterpart (which you saw on Marcy) into Boys and Girls High—the school on Fulton Street at the start of the walk.

The Nostrand Avenue A and C trains are one block ahead at Fulton.

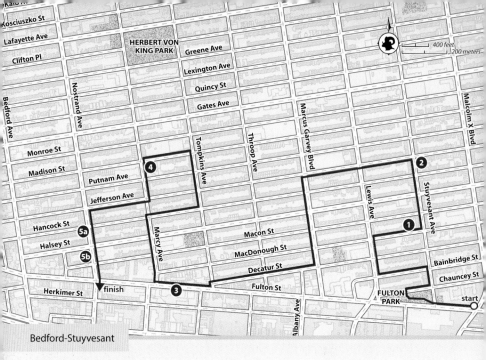

Points of Interest

1 **Akwaaba Mansion** 347 MacDonough St.; 866-466-3855, akwaaba.com

2 **Bridge Street AME Church** 277 Stuyvesant Ave.; 718-452-3936, bridgestreetbrooklyn.org

3 **Billie Holiday Theatre and Center for Arts & Culture** 1368 Fulton St.; 718-636-0918, thebillieholiday.org, restorationart.org

4 **Concord Baptist Church** 833 Marcy Ave.; 718-622-1818, concordcares.org

5 **Renaissance and Alhambra** 488 and 500–518 Nostrand Ave.

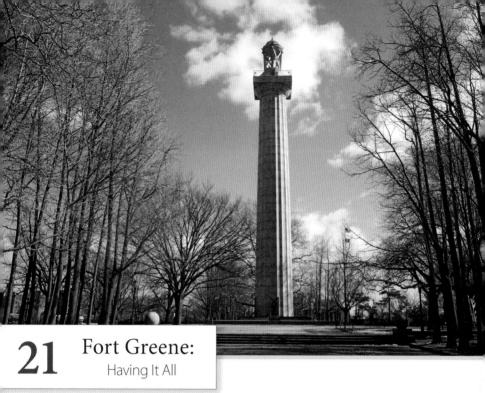

21 Fort Greene:
Having It All

Above: *The Prison Ship Martyrs Memorial in Fort Greene Park*

BOUNDARIES: Auburn Pl., Cumberland St., Hanson Pl., Flatbush Ave.
DISTANCE: 2.5 miles
SUBWAY: C to Lafayette Ave. (S. Oxford St. exit at Cuyler Gore)

Fort Greene is one of those Brooklyn neighborhoods where it's hard to go wrong. Want to see that quintessential Brooklyn streetscape? Fort Greene's got some of the finest blocks in the brownstone belt. Enjoy the arts? Not only is Fort Greene home to the country's oldest performing arts institution (the Brooklyn Academy of Music, or BAM), it also has professional theaters, art galleries, even entire buildings dedicated to providing artists of various genres with a place to flourish. Crave some fresh air? Fort Greene Park offers 30 acres of Olmsted and Vaux–designed greenery. History buff? The park took the place of a Revolutionary War fort, and atop its 105-foot hill stands a stirring memorial to the thousands who died aboard British prison ships in the Brooklyn harbor.

Fort Greene has a vibrant restaurant and retail scene too, as well as sites connected to cultural figures past and present. Plus, the neighborhood is a special source of pride for African Americans in many respects, from its cultural energy to its economic stability.

Walk Description

Follow signs in the subway to South Oxford Street and use the exit for Cuyler Gore. Feel free to pop into the park. Local abolitionist minister Theodore Ledyard Cuyler humbly declined to have a statue erected of himself here.

With your back to the park and the tall domed clocktower (the former Williamsburgh Savings Bank, featured on Walk 5) ahead of you, cross Fulton Street and head down Hanson Place to your left. After crossing South Oxford street, on your left will be Hanson Place Seventh Day Adventist Church, a city landmark completed in 1860, whose grandeur comes not just from its striking exterior—Corinthian columns and all—but from what took place out of sight of passersby: the property (under its original Baptist congregation) was part of the Underground Railroad.

Across South Portland Avenue, visit ❶ **MoCADA,** the Museum of Contemporary African Diasporan Arts. It is located in the 80 Arts Building, which offers affordable office space to arts-related organizations.

Cross Hanson Place and head north on South Portland Avenue. Upon reaching Fulton Street, don't overlook the lovely Neo-Renaissance apartment building from the turn of the century on your left, though your attention will probably be drawn to the mural on your right paying tribute to the Notorious B.I.G., the rapper who grew up in neighboring Clinton Hill. It's on a side of the Brooklyn Love Building, whose name is inspired by rapper Biggie's "Juicy" lyric "Spread love, it's the Brooklyn way." This building contains the take-out branch of Habana Outpost across Fulton. This "eco-eatery," which uses solar and wind power and has patio tables made out of recycled material, hosts film screenings, artisan markets, and other events.

Turn left on Fulton in front of ❷ **Greenlight Bookstore,** an amazing success story. It was opened by two young women in 2009, in the midst of the recession and the internet's decimation of brick-and-mortar bookstores, and has become an invaluable community resource, with author events, children's programming, book clubs, podcasts, and partnerships with local schools and cultural groups. Do take note of the street's namesake, Robert Fulton, in the painting above the door next to Greenlight, pictured along with one of the steam vessels he made possible.

Turn right onto the pedestrian plaza of South Elliott Place—a good place to photograph the Williamsburgh Savings Bank clocktower. General Fowler, on the west side of South Elliott, commanded a regiment at Bull Run, Gettysburg, and other major Civil War battles; lived just a couple of blocks away (and got married in a church on Hanson Place); and lay in state at Brooklyn's City Hall after his death. With Fowler to your left, you can see a red banner on South Elliott across Lafayette Avenue with 40A in a circle. That's the headquarters of 40 Acres and a Mule Filmworks, director Spike Lee's production company. Lee used to live in the neighborhood and shot his 1986 breakout film, *She's Gotta Have It,* in Fort Greene Park.

Make a right on Lafayette Avenue.

Turn left on South Portland Avenue, admiring the right-corner mansion from both its brownstone front on Lafayette and its brick side on South Portland with bilevel bay windows. Many of the South Portland homes—which date mostly to the late 1860s and 1870s—were built in groups of two to five, giving the street a uniform look with just a few exceptions. Those include the 1850s brick homes from #72 to #62 and the refaced frame house at #60, which is likely the oldest on the block (circa 1852).

Turn right on DeKalb Avenue and then right on South Oxford Street. While it has brick and brownstone rowhouses similar in age and style to those on South Portland, it's a more varied block, and a few of its apartment buildings come with interesting backstories. Take, for example, the limestone building partway down on your right with L-shaped stoop and oval windows. Its right half was built in the 1850s in tandem with the brick house next door; its left half was built in 1879 as part of a row with the two brownstones on that side. In 1893 the formerly separate houses were combined into one grand residence—since subdivided into apartments—and remodeled in the front by Montrose Morris, a premier architect of the time.

Morris is also the presumed architect of the Roanoke, down the block on the left, an early-1890s Romanesque design distinguished by a curving front stoop and bay windows. It stands opposite the Griffin, an Art Deco former hotel from the early 1930s. Look for the half-bird, half-lion creature for which it's named around the door and at the corner, peering across Lafayette Avenue at the church with the tall brown tower. This is Lafayette Avenue Presbyterian Church, where Reverend Cuyler—remember the gore?—was pastor for its first 30 years. It was a stop on the Underground Railroad and has remained involved in social-justice issues to this day. Cuyler was known nationwide (even by Abraham Lincoln) for his antislavery activism but nonetheless was censured by Presbyterian authorities for inviting a woman to preach at the church. When Sarah Smiley, a Quaker, addressed the LAPC congregation in 1872, she became the first woman ever to preach from a Presbyterian pulpit. St. Paul was given Reverend Cuyler's face in the church's Tiffany stained-glass windows. A church hall, entered on South Oxford, has been converted to an off-Broadway theater, the Irondale Center, complete with a same-named resident company.

Turn left on Lafayette Avenue facing the church.

Make a left on Cumberland Street. This eclectic block features a converted church; the long-time home of a Pulitzer Prize–winning poet (read the plaque at #260 about how much Marianne Moore, a native Missourian, loved Brooklyn); and well-preserved frame houses of the early 1850s at #252, 243, and 235. Across DeKalb, the street takes the name Washington Park, a former name of the actual park on your left. A few steps along, you can see the top of the Prison Ship Martyrs Memorial in the park, a monument that honors the approximately 11,500 prisoners of war who perished during the Revolutionary War aboard British ships docked in Wallabout Bay (which was landfilled to build the Brooklyn Navy Yard)—a death toll almost three times as great as the war's combat casualties. You will soon get up close to the memorial, but first, enjoy this splendid brownstone block of Washington Park.

Enter ❸ **Fort Greene Park** opposite Willoughby Avenue. Go to the right, staying on the path as it curves left, then right again en route to the visitor center, housed in a 1908 mini-temple that may have been the last thing designed by architect Stanford White before the famed architect was murdered by his mistress's husband in one of the city's all-time most-buzzed-about scandals. Exhibits inside focus on the park's birds and trees and Revolutionary War history (the cannons, though, are Civil War surplus). The redoubt of Fort Putnam, which preceded the park on this site, has been re-created next to the visitor center.

Proceed to the Prison Ship Martyrs Memorial, which was *definitely* designed by Stanford White. The world's highest (150 feet) freestanding Doric column supports an eight-ton bronze urn—originally lit by oil but outfitted, after years of darkness, with LED lighting in the memorial's centennial renovation in 2008.

Continue past the memorial to the plaza (down steps) on the other side. Back around 1939, you might have encountered a diligent young man here in the early morning—Richard Wright, working on a Chicago-set story the world would later know as *Native Son*. Wright lived a block away (at 175 Carlton Ave.) but preferred writing on the hill from 6 to 10 a.m. Head to the bench at the far end of the plaza to see Wright's words imprinted on its legs.

When you're walking back toward the Prison Ship Martyrs monument, the large trees with whiter trunks on your left are 150-year-old London planes, planted here in the formal design for the park by landscape architects Frederick Law Olmsted and Calvert Vaux (implemented in 1867, following the pair's success with Central Park). The park had been established in 1847 after campaigning by *Brooklyn Eagle* editor Walt Whitman, who was concerned about ample breathing room for crowded city dwellers.

Now head down the broad staircase. Inset in the middle of it is a crypt containing some of the prison-ship victims' remains. Go straight at the bottom of the steps, then turn right at the basketball courts, and follow the path to the park exit on Myrtle Avenue at North Portland Avenue.

Cross Myrtle and walk on North Portland to Auburn Place, where you turn left. The elegant structure on your right was built in 1920 for Cumberland Hospital—which traces its origins to 1851, when it was founded as the City of Brooklyn's first public hospital. Basketball great Michael Jordan was born at Cumberland in 1963. Bernard King, also a basketball hall of famer and contemporary of Jordan, was born here, too, as was boxer Mike Tyson.

Proceed on Auburn to St. Edwards Street, opposite the shuttered St. Michael and St. Edward Church. To your right is the one branch of the Brooklyn Public Library that carries the name of the greatest literary figure associated with the borough, Walt Whitman. The brick building dates to 1907 and was paid for by Andrew Carnegie. P.S. 67, next to the library, is where formal education began for the black population of Brooklyn. It opened in 1847 as Colored School No. 1, serving a student body composed of the children of freed slaves, many of whom were employed at the Brooklyn Navy Yard, located just a few blocks north. The two housing projects on either side of St. Edwards Street—together comprising some 3,500 apartments—were built by the city for World War II–era employees of the Navy Yard.

Turn left from Auburn onto St. Edwards. Cross Myrtle Avenue, walking beside the park. Ahead you see the radio tower (and building) of Brooklyn Tech, a prestigious admission-by-exam public high school. Turn right on Willoughby Street next to the Brooklyn Hospital Center.

Make a left on Ashland Place, with the LIU (Long Island University) athletic facilities to your right and the Williamsburgh Savings Bank tower ahead of you. For the first 80 years of its existence, the 512-foot-tall clocktower (now a luxury condo) was described as Brooklyn's only skyscraper. Not so anymore. Make a 180-degree turn and you'll see the Empire State Building, which no longer ranks tallest in its borough either.

From Ashland, turn right on Fulton Street to encounter a succession of creative enterprises. First is the BAM Harvey Theater (named for BAM's former executive director Harvey Lichtenstein), still displaying its earlier name, Majestic, because when BAM took over the 1903 theater, it restored but did not overlay any part of its exterior or interior. The main building of BAM, the Brooklyn Academy of Music, is a block down Ashland (and featured on Walk 5), but the performing arts institution—founded in 1859 in Brooklyn Heights—has been expanding its footprint in the 21st century.

Next to the BAM Harvey, visit the Agnes Varis Art Center, where a store and gallery showcase glass objets d'art. ❹ **Urban Glass,** which runs the center, also offers classes and studios for those using glass as their creative medium. The public can take studio tours on the weekend. It's all located within ❺ **BRIC House,** another old theater restored and adapted for use by an arts organization. Turn right onto Rockwell Place and enter this home of BRIC (Brooklyn Information & Culture), where you're welcome to hang out at the café and in the Stoop, the tiered public space on the ground floor. BRIC House also contains a gallery, a large performance space known as the Ballroom, a black-box theater, a cable-access TV studio, classrooms, and artist workspace.

Turn left on DeKalb Avenue, walking with the LIU Brooklyn campus on your right. Watch for an aerial bridge between two buildings—then examine the side of the building on the left end of the bridge. Can you make out the Paramount's name in cursive above the school banners and terra cotta rosettes and masks of comedy? The 4,000-seat Paramount, at the corner of DeKalb and Flatbush Avenue, thrived from 1928 to 1962, before cookie-cutter multiplexes displaced opulent movie palaces. People flocked to the theater not just for movies but also live shows: everyone from Ethel Merman to Miles Davis to Frank Sinatra performed on the Paramount stage, and in the '50s deejay Alan Freed presented the first-ever rock and roll concerts here. For years LIU basketball fans watched games in a gymnasium with a carved wood ceiling and Wurlitzer organ, both of which the school had preserved when it converted the theater. It also incorporated the theater's two-story lobby, with grand staircase, columns, and marble walls, into the student center. In 2016 LIU signed a deal with the developer of the Barclays Center to renovate the Paramount and reopen it as a venue for concerts and other performances as well as boxing matches. The reborn Brooklyn Paramount is scheduled to debut in 2019.

Wrap up your walk as Paramount theatergoers used to wrap up their evenings: with a bite at ❻ **Junior's,** across Flatbush Avenue. Beloved for its cheesecake, Junior's is also good for classic New York fare like matzo ball soup, pastrami sandwiches, and blintzes—though its huge menu covers plenty more. The restaurant has been holding strong at this location since 1950. There are entrances to the B/D/Q/R DeKalb Avenue subway station on both sides of Flatbush.

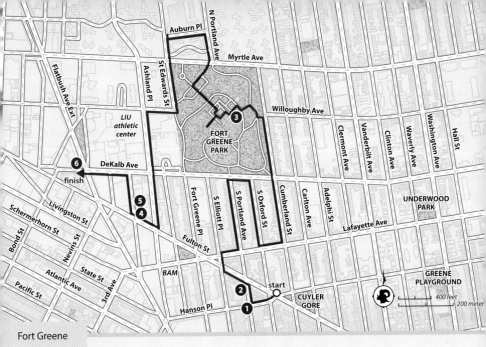

Fort Greene

Points of Interest

1. **MoCADA** 80 Hanson Place; 718-230-0492, mocada.org
2. **Greenlight Bookstore** 686 Fulton St.; 718-246-0200, greenlightbookstore.com
3. **Fort Greene Park** Washington Park and Willoughby Avenue; 718-722-3218, fortgreenepark.org
4. **Urban Glass** 647 Fulton St.; 718-625-3685, urbanglass.org
5. **BRIC House** Rockwell Place and Fulton Street; 718-683-5600, bricartsmedia.org
6. **Junior's** 386 Flatbush Ave. Extension; 718-852-5257, juniorscheesecake.com

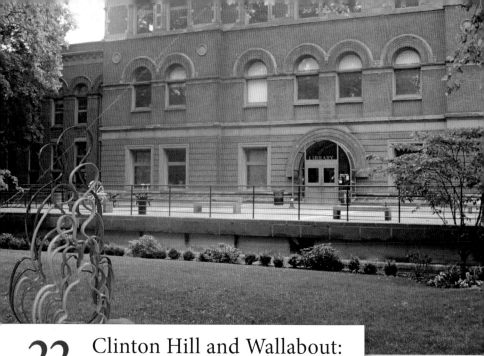

22 Clinton Hill and Wallabout:
Posh Enclave Turned College Town

Above: Pratt Institute's campus is a sculpture park, and the college offers a sculpture major too

BOUNDARIES: Park Ave., Classon Ave., Gates Ave., Vanderbilt Ave.
DISTANCE: 2.9 miles, plus .75-mile optional extension
SUBWAY: G to Classon Ave.

In the late 19th century, Clinton Hill was the most prestigious address in Brooklyn after Brooklyn Heights. Charles Pratt, Brooklyn's wealthiest resident and the owner of Greenpoint-based Astral Oil, put the neighborhood on the map when he moved into his brand-new mansion in 1875. Pratt's fellow tycoons, some of whose names we know today from the companies they founded, followed Pratt to "The Hill"—among them, Messrs. Pfizer, Bristol, and Liebmann (owner of Rhein-gold brewery). Pratt helped fund other construction in the area, including speculative housing on the block of Vanderbilt Avenue that's now the Wallabout Historic District. Wallabout started losing its identity as a neighborhood discrete from Clinton Hill when production dwindled at the Brooklyn Navy Yard and local factories after World War II, but the name's been revived of late, as the area north of Myrtle Avenue has become desirable to developers, retailers, and residents.

Walk Description

With the playground at Classon and Lafayette Avenues to your left, walk north on Classon. On your left at the corner with DeKalb Avenue is the NYPD's 88th Precinct, housed in a landmarked 1890 brick building with a high conical tower.

Turn left from Classon onto Willoughby Avenue. What you see at the corner of Classon and Willoughby on your right depends on how far St. Mary's Episcopal Church has proceeded with plans to demolish its 19th-century rectory and replace it with a 16-story apartment building. The church itself isn't going anywhere, and you have a good view of the green-steepled Gothic Revival landmark (1859) from Willoughby when you're halfway down the block.

At Emerson Place, look to your left at the rowhouses that make a U-formation with rows fronting Willoughby and Steuben, the next cross street. There are 27 houses in all, built in 1907 for faculty of Pratt Institute and presenting such picturesque features as alternating stepped and triangular gables and three-sided, two-story bays with diamond-pane windows. The university has been renovating them for student dorms.

Past Steuben Street, enter ❶ **Pratt Institute** through its main gate, and follow Grand Walk. Charles Pratt founded this design and engineering college, whose campus doubles as a top-notch sculpture park.

On your right after the Student Union stands one of the first buildings constructed for the school. Now called the East Building and formerly known as the Machine Shop—note the smokestack—it contains the oldest steam-powered generators still in use in the Northeast. Go into the building through the door with an intertwined *P* and *I* above it for a look at this extraordinary power plant, which served as a laboratory for Pratt's engineering students in the early days and still provides heat and hot water for the campus. You'll also see assorted obsolete industrial pieces and, perhaps, a display of cat-show ribbons. The cats that won them, plus a bunch of their compadres, used to roam this building freely; they were the famous Pratt Cats, strays taken in and fed by the chief engineer who ran the steam plant for 58 years.

Exit the building on the other end of the corridor from where you came in. You'll be in a courtyard with a trickling fountain carved with a forest scene and mythological figures. Take the steps to your left, which lead through the semicircular bleachers of a small amphitheater.

Facing a lawn arrayed with sculptures, go to the right. On your right at Ryerson Walk are three adjoining Romanesque edifices. The Main Building in the middle, like the Machine Shop, opened with the school in 1887. A few years later came South Hall, whose architect then created the porch for the Main Building. Memorial Hall was added to the campus in the 1920s.

Cross Ryerson Walk from the Main Building. Up a few steps you'll find a rose garden—most noticeable, obviously, when it's in bloom. Pratt's library, an 1896 building to your left, was originally a public library—the first free one in Brooklyn, in fact. Walk on the path beside the library, coming around to its entrance. In front of the library, a lawn of sculptures encircles Cannon Plaza. This bronze cannon was cast in Spain in the 1720s (hence the insignia of King Philip V, the Spanish monarch at the time) and had been installed at Morro Castle in Havana Bay, Cuba, before the college acquired it.

Return to Grand Walk, then head north back to the gate where you entered.

Turn left on Willoughby Avenue. Before turning left at Washington Avenue, get a glimpse of the magnificent double mansion on Washington to your right, built in 1892 for the Van Glahn brothers, whose name can still be seen on their former grocery warehouse in Wallabout.

Make a left on Washington and head south. Down the block on your left, St. Luke's Church was purchased for conversion to condos in 2015. This side of the street also has a couple of the oldest freestanding houses in the neighborhood: the brownstone mansion (1873) next to the former church and, four doors past that, an Italianate villa (1865) with wraparound porch. Opposite the latter is a grand composition from 1887: twin townhouses with curving stoops and second-floor arched loggias. The picturesque Queen Anne trio at the end of the block on your left was designed to look like one big house.

Cross DeKalb Avenue and take note on your right of #320, an apartment building still inscribed GRAHAM HOME FOR OLD LADIES—a now laughably insensitive name that reveals only part of the place's history. After operating for more than a century in its original capacity, it deteriorated into a flophouse occupied by other kinds of ladies (of the evening) and was later a squalid welfare hotel, but it's been restored as co-op apartments. Next to it, Underwood Park is named for the typewriter mogul whose mansion once stood here and whose widow donated the land to the city.

Before proceeding to the next block, check out the side-by-side houses of worship to your left on Lafayette Avenue. Apostolic Faith Church occupies a former Orthodox Friends meetinghouse, built in 1868 following the schism in Quakerism that resulted in two sects (the Orthodox one broke with tradition by employing a pastor). The French Gothic masterpiece ❷ **Emmanuel Baptist Church,** constructed in 1887, was paid for by Charles Pratt, a devout Baptist. You should see its St. James Place side, too, and its interior, if possible.

Return to Washington south of Lafayette. The first two pairs on both sides date to 1861–63. Next up on the left is a lovely brick manse (1888) with peak-roofed dormer and a balustrade atop the bay window. The home adjoining it on the right was built 20 years later for Mr. Bristol of pharmaceutical fame (his factory was also in the neighborhood). The second half of the block on the left consists of the buildings of the Mohawk. The shorter ones were built in 1904 as an extension to the Beaux Arts #379, opened in 1903 as a fashionable residential hotel. The property declined into seediness and then was shuttered for more than a decade before being renovated as apartments in the 1980s. Completing this impressive block on your right is a group of Queen Anne stunners, originally five separate houses constructed 1885–87. Try to make out the expressive faun faces in the terra cotta panel beneath the top window of #400. Turn right on Greene Avenue, where you see other delightful features of the corner property.

Turn left on Clinton Avenue. The elegant lampposts in front of #385 warrant a few moments of your time. Then pass another apartment building before you encounter a number of superb freestanding houses. The star of the show is #405, built in 1889 by a preeminent architect of the time, William Tubby, for a preeminent citizen of the time, Charles A. Schieren—a leather magnate who served a term as mayor of Brooklyn. You wouldn't think the word *quaint* goes with $6.5 million (the home's 2014 sales price), but that's certainly an apt description for the bottleneck-shaped gable, pyramidal-roofed dormer, fish-scale roof tiles, and other distinctive features of this house. Another marquee name in Victorian-age architecture, the Parfitt Brothers, are represented across the street with the wonderful Queen Anne at #410. The block's panoply of styles encompasses neo-Jacobean, #443; French Second Empire, #457; and Beaux Arts, #463–465.

Make a right on Gates Avenue. The ❸ **Royal Castle** on your left is brimming with character. Characters, actually—see the figures "holding up" the central bays, and if you can make out what's at the top corners, you'll see guys with creepy faces giving thumbs-up with both hands. This landmark built around 1911 still rates as one of the city's finest old apartment houses.

Turn right on Vanderbilt Avenue. A long row of 1880s Italianate brownstones stretches out on your left.

Go left at Lafayette Avenue for a good look at two ornate structures on the north side: the column-fronted Brooklyn Masonic Temple, admired for its terra cotta detail, and Queen of All Saints church, with over 20 statues.

Turn around and head in the other direction on Lafayette. On the right corner across Vanderbilt is a yellow clapboard house with shutters and an octagonal cupola. Its smaller eastern wing may look like an annex, but that section dates to 1812, while the rest of it is from the 1850s. This landmark is variously known as the ❹ **Joseph Steele or Steele–Brick–Skinner house,** depending on how many previous owners you wish to cite.

Turn left on Clinton. Some houses here are considered the neighborhood's finest sampling of their respective styles: #324 for Second French Empire; #315, Romanesque; and #313, Neo-Grec. All three were constructed in the 1880s for owners of major manufacturing concerns—respectively, pottery, coffee, and lace. Cross DeKalb, and past the apartment building on your left is a shingled chalet from the mid-1850s, followed by the quirky #278, with its two types of windows and two different balconies. Then you approach the ❺ **Pratt homes,** some of them now used by St. Joseph's College. On the right are three mansions that Charles Pratt had built for his sons as wedding presents: the Georgian-style #245 was the last to go up, in 1901; #241, designed by William Tubby, was the first in 1890 (and today is the Roman Catholic bishop of Brooklyn's residence); the palazzo at #229, featuring a two-story portico whose upper-level columns bear busts, became the home of Pratt Institute's president. As for pater Pratt, he lived at #232 across the street.

Across Willoughby, another splendid Clinton Avenue residence has its own father-son connection. Head to the limestone extravaganza at #186–184, a double house built for two William Beards: the father, who owned a dredging company (the Navy Yard was a client) and was active in politics, and his elder son. But Beard senior never got to live here: he died in 1893 while the home was under construction. The architect was Montrose Morris, who also designed large double houses with prominent corner towers in Park Slope and Crown Heights.

Two groups of commanding brick-and-brownstone buildings fill out the block on the left side, with the corner structure capped by a conical roof. It has a bank at street level, just as it did when the building opened in 1888 as the Wallabout Bank's main branch. Novelist Henry Miller, a Brooklyn native, lived at 180 Clinton Ave. for a while; he later wrote in *Tropic of Capricorn,* "you must see Myrtle Avenue before you die, if only to realize how far into the future Dante saw. It is a street not of sorrow . . . but of sheer emptiness . . . ."

With that, cross Myrtle, but go only as far as the two landmarked residences side-by-side on your left. The "temple front" was common when the ❻ **Lefferts-Laidlaw House,** as #136 is known, was built in the late 1830s, but today it's the only Greek Revival house left in Brooklyn that looks like this. As a clapboard-covered wood-frame dwelling, #128 was also typical of its period (1853–54), but today it's atypically well preserved for this type of home. Which type is that? Well, the columned porch, among other features, is Italianate in style, but the columns themselves— fluted, with Corinthian capitals—would be classified Greek Revival.

Return to Myrtle Avenue, make a right, and then take a right onto Vanderbilt Avenue. The Wallabout Historic District, designated in 2011, is confined to this block and composed primarily of wood-frame houses built between 1849 and 1855. There are also a few brick or brownstone flats buildings and rowhouses from the 1870s and 1880s, as well as a recent construction (#118) that shows you where the neighborhood is headed. In addition to its architecture, the historic district was designated for its link to Brooklyn's maritime heritage: harbor pilots resided at #117 and 123, a boatswain at #102, a ship captain at #121, and ferrymen at #128. Meanwhile, #124 and 110 are among the 1850s houses that were gussied up in the 1870s with the addition of a third floor and fish-scale shingling.

From Park Avenue, you can walk back to Clinton and Lafayette for the G train (or take the bus on Vanderbilt to Lafayette) or continue through industrial Wallabout to the Brooklyn Navy Yard, as detailed below.

Extension

The Navy Yard sits on Wallabout Bay, which had the name before the neighborhood; it apparently evolved from *Walloons*—French people from Belgium, who'd settled there in the 17th century.

Turn right on Park Avenue. To your right on Clinton Avenue, opposite a few old frame houses, #77 is currently used by Benjamin Banneker Academy but was erected in 1913 for Drake's bakery, when it was still just making pound cake—Yodels, Ring Dings, and Devil Dogs would be invented in this building before Drake's moved out in the late '60s.

Wallabout has something of a sweet (fattening?) heritage: across Park Avenue, the building spanning Clinton to Waverly Avenue was built in 1915 for a cookie and cracker factory. Go one more block on that side of Park Avenue, and that's where Rockwood & Co. ran the country's second-largest chocolate factory. Look for the corner building at Washington Avenue with a cursive VAN GLAHN BROS. embossed on a panel above the door. Rockwood acquired the building from the Van Glahn grocery wholesalers in 1904 and proceeded to add 15 more buildings to its complex.

A significant non-confectionery operation in Wallabout was Mergenthaler Linotype, whose property one block away is now the Hall Street Industrial Complex. Mergenthaler invented the linotype machine, which mechanized typesetting and would be adopted by almost every newspaper. From here, you can proceed east to a new Navy Yard green space off of Flushing Avenue and Steuben Street (see last paragraph of the sidebar on the next page), or turn around and head west for the museum and visitor center and food hall. If you choose the latter, take Park Avenue back to Vanderbilt and make a right. The block from Park to Flushing Avenue contains two new residential developments: a bright red building of studio apartments, and then the Navy Green townhouses. There are also a couple of new food and drink spots at the north end on the right. Go left on Flushing to the Navy Yard's Building 77 or 92 (see sidebar).

Brooklyn Navy Yard

The Brooklyn Navy Yard, once the borough's largest employer with a World War II–era workforce of 70,000, has become a leisure-time destination. A rooftop wine garden, historic museum, and distillery and cocktail bar are some of the new public amenities at the Navy Yard, which ceased its original operations in 1966. The Navy Yard was converted to an industrial park not long after its military decommissioning, and many tenants are engaged in creative industries, like fashion design, antique-furniture restoration, woodworking, jewelry making, and set construction. It's also home to several artist's' workshops, as well as Steiner Studios, the largest television and film production complex outside Hollywood.

Buildings 77 and 92—key visitor destinations—both have entrances on Flushing Avenue. **BLDG 92,** the museum and visitor center, is opposite Carlton Avenue (63 Flushing Ave.; 718-907-5992, bldg92.org). Its three-level exhibition takes you through the entire history of the Navy Yard, illustrated with artifacts that include a relic from the USS *Arizona,* the battleship destroyed at Pearl Harbor that had been built at the Navy Yard, and a model of the USS *Missouri,* also built at the Navy Yard, just a few years before Japan signed the surrender aboard it to end WWII. One section of the museum highlights products currently manufactured at the Navy Yard. BLDG 92 is also the starting point for the superb guided tour "Past, Present & Future"— hopping on and off a tour bus, you visit locales throughout the yard, including its still-active dry docks, for a comprehensive survey of all that has happened and is planned there. The trip is operated by **Turnstile Tours** (347-903-8687, turnstiletours.com), which also offers themed Navy Yard tours focusing on sustainable architecture and industry or showcasing on-site businesses, where you get to meet artisans and entrepreneurs.

The Navy Yard's Building 77, at Vanderbilt Avenue, contains a new food hall anchored by the first outer-borough location of Lower East Side smoked-fish emporium Russ & Daughters. Its eateries specialize in Korean barbecue, West Indian stews, chocolate, coffee, and more. Situated between BLDG 92 and the food hall is the building with Brooklyn Grange, a 1.5-acre rooftop farm. Open to the public only for a weekly tour, Brooklyn Grange is a commercial fruit and vegetable farm that also provides environmental benefits like insulating the building and absorbing rainwater.

Wine and spirits drinkers should visit Rooftop Reds and Kings County Distillery, which are accessed from the Navy Yard's Sands Street gate in Dumbo (see Walk 3). Meanwhile, all the way on the far east side of the Navy Yard is a small new park called the **Naval Cemetery Landscape.** Don't be scared away from this unique oasis by the name. The site *was* the burial ground for the Navy Yard hospital, but only until 1910, and many of those buried there were reinterred at Cypress Hills Cemetery back in the 1920s. Now it's a wildflower meadow ringed by tall, lush trees and traversed via an elevated boardwalk. The entrance is just north of Flushing Avenue on Williamsburg Street West, near Steuben Street

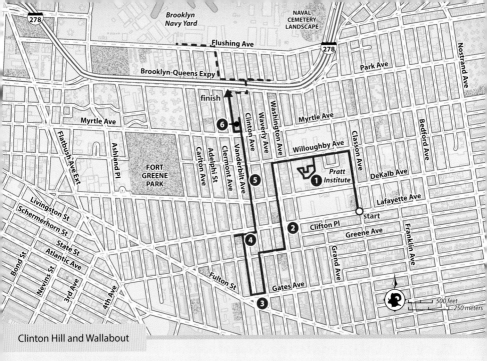

Points of Interest

1 Pratt Institute 200 Willoughby Ave.; 718-636-3600, pratt.edu

2 Emmanuel Baptist Church 279 Lafayette Ave.; 718-622-1107, ebcconnects.com

3 Royal Castle 20–30 Gates Ave.

4 Joseph Steele (Steele–Brick–Skinner) House 200 Lafayette Ave.

5 Pratt family mansions 229, 232, 241, 245 Clinton Ave.

6 Lefferts-Laidlaw House 136 Clinton Ave.

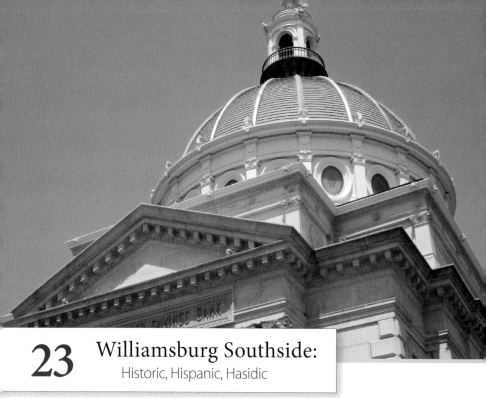

23 Williamsburg Southside:
Historic, Hispanic, Hasidic

Above: *The Williamsburgh Savings Bank erected this building resembling Florence's Duomo as its headquarters in 1875*

BOUNDARIES: S. 4th St., Hewes St., Bedford Ave., Berry St.
DISTANCE: 2.9 miles
SUBWAY: J, M, or Z to Marcy Ave. (Havemeyer St. exit)

Williamsburg went through many identities on its way to becoming the worldwide paragon of a trendsetting, artisanal lifestyle. From a farming village in the 17th-century Dutch settlement of Boswijck (Bushwick), it eventually grew into a center of brewing and manufacturing, and by 1852 was large enough to charter as a city. But three years later Williamsburgh (as it was spelled then) lost its independence, and the *h* at the end of its name, when annexed by the city of Brooklyn. Then its days as a well-off suburb and resort came to an end with the opening of the Williamsburg Bridge in 1903. Immigrants crowded out of Manhattan's Lower East Side, directly across the river,

142 Williamsburg Southside

began to crowd into tenements in Williamsburg—an era depicted in *A Tree Grows in Brooklyn*. New immigrant communities arose after World War II: first Hasidic Jews from Eastern Europe, and later Puerto Ricans and other Hispanics. Both groups reside on the south side, or "Los Sures" to Latinos.

Note: *You can precede or conclude this tour with a walk across the Williamsburg Bridge. Look for the pedestrian-access ramp on Bedford Avenue between South 5th and South 6th Streets—roughly five blocks from the tour's starting and ending point.*

Walk Description

Down the stairs from the train, walk straight ahead on Broadway and make a right on Havemeyer Street. The Havemeyers ran a sugar company in Williamsburg—the one we know today as Domino. At one time, nearly all sugar consumed in the United States was produced in Brooklyn. Domino was the last major sugar company operating here; the 11-acre spread under the Williamsburg Bridge that it vacated in 2004 is currently being redeveloped.

Across South 5th Street on your right, the Dime Savings Bank's former headquarters is due to be incorporated into a new 22-story building that will stretch almost to South 4th Street.

Turn left on South 4th Street, steering clear of the vehicle-access lanes for the Williamsburg Bridge. On your right at Roebling Street, a former church building is the flagship location of El Puente, an advocacy and education organization that grew out of an anti-gang-violence initiative of the early '80s. Its cultural center in this building includes a dance studio, theater, and art room.

Cross over to ❶ **Continental Army Plaza** kitty-corner from El Puente, and come around to the front of the statue of George Washington on horseback at Valley Forge. The sculptor chose not to glorify triumph in war but to honor a warrior's fortitude: Washington is swathed in a blanket, and his horse also looks worn down by the arduous wintertime campaign.

Cross South 5th Place to the beautiful domed structure erected in 1906 by the Williamsburgh Trust Company. Bearing full temple fronts on two sides, the building is dappled with floral- and shell-shaped ornamentation and faced in white terra cotta. Just one year after the building opened, the bank closed amid a financial crisis (and its owners' conspiracy indictments). The building was a courthouse from 1916 to 1958—conveniently, Lady Justice is featured in the bank's seal, above the doors—and acquired in the early '60s by the Eastern Orthodox church that still occupies it.

With the former bank on your right, walk on South 5th Street, then turn left on Driggs Avenue and walk under the bridge to Broadway. Go left for a full look at the fine cast-iron edifice on this corner, built as a shoe warehouse in 1882. See how the Forman shoemakers marked their territory with both letters and a 4MAN logo. Then turn your attention to the domed gem across Driggs, erected in 1875 for the Williamsburgh Savings Bank. Its initials—etched in glass panes around the base of the 110-foot dome—were adapted for the tony event venue now here, ❷ **Weylin B. Seymour's.** The opulent interior features a mosaic marble floor and stained-glass skylight; the exterior is richly detailed too, right down to the lampposts. Another Williamsburg icon is directly across Broadway, legendary steakhouse Peter Luger. It originated in 1876 as a billiards café and bowling alley and in 1887 became a restaurant that served *only* porterhouse steak—not even any veggies on the side. The menu has diversified, though porterhouse remains its raison d'être.

Head down Broadway with Peter Luger on your left. At the next intersection, Bedford Avenue, another magnificent former bank stands on your right. This 1868 French Second Empire landmark boasts a tiled mansard roof that tells you who built it (see it from Bedford): the Kings County Savings Bank. The ❸ **Williamsburg Art & Historical (WAH) Center,** a pioneering proponent of the local arts scene, was founded in this building in 1996 and still maintains galleries inside.

There's some craftsmanship to be admired on the other side of Broadway too. The 1882 cast-iron building opposite the WAH Center was originally a department store and now holds residential lofts. On the southwest corner with Bedford, the balustraded and columned Renaissance palazzo, designed by the same architect as the white-domed former bank next to the bridge, was built in 1901 for yet another defunct financial institution.

Go onto South 6th Street, also branching off from Bedford Avenue. The brick building on your right, a restored former theater, has a top floor of arched windows above facade medallions.

Turn left on Berry Street. That large gray building facing you to the right on Broadway is the former Gretsch musical instrument factory (now a luxury condo). Cross Broadway and enjoy the extravagantly ornamented old apartment building on your left.

Turn left on South 9th Street, which has gained a Hasidic presence as that population spread north of Division Avenue. Epiphany Roman Catholic Church, on your right, has served Williamsburg's Hispanic population as a civic voice and cultural center as well as house of worship. Don't miss the terra cotta–rich 1880s apartment house opposite it.

The playground across Bedford is tied up in history with Schaefer beer. The brewery traded this parcel to the city in the 1950s for a former ferry landing five blocks away, allowing Schaefer (the last Brooklyn brewery to close, in 1976) to expand its waterfront plant. There's an elegant apartment building at the end of the block on the left—look at its Driggs side as you cross the avenue.

Watch on your left for the landmark ❹ **New England Congregational Church,** but don't expect the Congregationalists' traditional white exterior and spire. Founded in 1853, the church had to be rebuilt after an 1890s fire, and it later passed through Lutheran hands before becoming a Spanish-speaking Pentecostal house, La Luz del Mundo, in 1955.

Turn right on Roebling Street, right on Division Avenue, then left on Clymer Street, beneath one of several huge buildings the Hasids have constructed or redeveloped in the neighborhood.

Make a left on Bedford, a moneyed avenue at the turn of the century. The Second Empire house at #499 may be Bedford's oldest, built as early as the 1870s. Jewish youth now attend school in mansions where the WASP upper crust used to gather. For instance, #499 served as the Breevort Club for a while, while the Congress Club met in #505 (it was built in 1896 for a sugar magnate). A couple of blocks farther, the street's most opulent mansion commands the corner of Rodney, with its bulbous tower, loggia, and terra cotta aplenty. It was built for the owners of the store whose cast-iron building you saw at Broadway and Bedford. Across Rodney Street, #563 dates to 1875, while #571 is completely different from its fellow Bedford mansions and perhaps the most dramatic.

All these streets you've passed since turning onto Bedford were named after signers of the Declaration of Independence. Williamsburg has 27 such streets in all, including the next cross street, Keap. Its namesake was actually Thomas McKean, but his signature was misread as Thomas M. Keap by town planners and the error never corrected. After Keap, cross the Brooklyn-Queens Expressway (BQE). About 5,000 Williamsburg residents were displaced by its construction in the early 1950s.

Turn left from Bedford onto Hewes Street and then left on Marcy, in front of Transfiguration Roman Catholic Church, here since 1875. The community outreach of this Latino parish (originally Irish and German) includes services for the homeless, people with HIV, and undocumented immigrants. Go another block on Marcy, and at Keap Street behold the grimy Gothic glory of the former ❺ **Eastern District High School** to your right. Alumni include Mel Brooks, Barry Manilow, Red Auerbach, Joseph Papp, and Henry Miller. Cross Keap so you can take in all of the Marcy side.

Walk on Keap Street next to the school. At the end of the block on your right is the second-oldest synagogue in Brooklyn, built in 1876 by the oldest Jewish congregation in Brooklyn—a Reform congregation now based in a different neighborhood. Today the building is used by a Hasidic school.

Turn left on Division, then left on Rodney to pass the rounded rear of the local branch of the ❻ **Brooklyn Public Library.** Turn right on Marcy, then right on Division to come around to the front and see how it sits like an open book on this triangular plot. The library's old but not old enough to explain the "Williamsburgh" spelling. When it was built in 1905—Andrew Carnegie's second library endowment in Brooklyn—Williamsburg had been without its *h* for several decades.

Make a left back onto Rodney Street, walking under the elevated train toward the former St. Paul's Evangelical Lutheran Church, with its prominent belltower. See this 1885 landmark, designed by the architect of the Museum of Natural History in Manhattan, from both sides, then walk on South 5th past the playground and across the BQE overpass.

Go left on Marcy to Broadway, back at the subway station where you arrived.

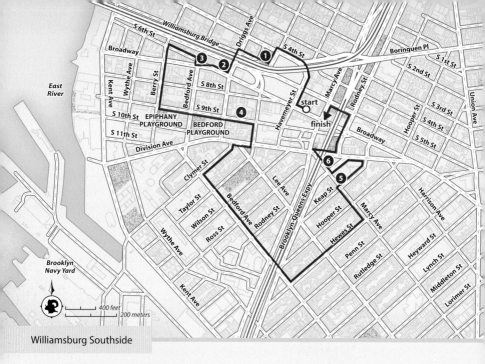

Williamsburg Southside

Points of Interest

1. **Continental Army Plaza** South 4th Street and South 5th Place; nycgovparks.org
2. **Weylin B. Seymour's (Williamsburgh Savings Bank)** 175 Broadway; 718-963-3639, weylin.com
3. **Williamsburg Art & Historical Center** 135 Broadway; 718-486-7372, wahcenter.net
4. **New England Congregational Church (now La Luz del Mundo)** 179 S. 9th St.
5. **Eastern District High School (former)** Marcy Avenue and Keap Street
6. **Brooklyn Public Library–Williamsburgh** 240 Division Ave., 718-302-3485, bklynlibrary.org /locations/williamsburgh

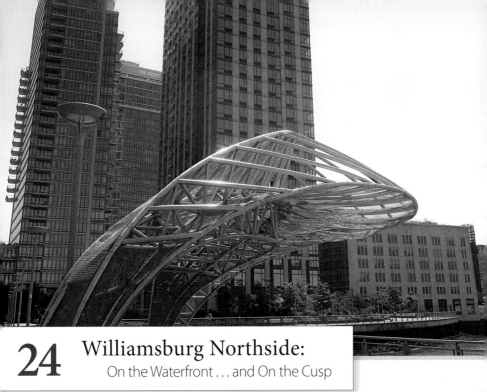

24 Williamsburg Northside:
On the Waterfront . . . and On the Cusp

Above: The Austin Nichols warehouse–turned–condo (right) was built in 1914, about 100 years before these other riverfront structures

BOUNDARIES: McCarren Park, Leonard St., Grand St., East River
DISTANCE: 3.9 miles
SUBWAY: L or G to Metropolitan Ave./Lorimer St. (Union Ave. exit)

As Florence, Italy, is to the Renaissance, Williamsburg's north side is to the Brooklyn renaissance: where it all began. In the 1990s, artists who couldn't afford the East Village discovered the area. That paved the way for an influx of white middle-class college grads with bohemian aspirations. Before you knew it, no one could get through a sentence about Williamsburg without using the word *hipster*—and this sprawling, historic neighborhood vaulted to the forefront of real estate interest, culinary trends, indie art and music, and other creative pursuits. Meanwhile, gentrification and artisanal ideals spread to other Brooklyn neighborhoods. Some people may tell you the old

Williamsburg—ethnic, industrial, modestly scaled—has been totally erased, but you'll discover that's not true on this walk, which also shows you a sampling of the innovative enterprises, tasty treats, and pricey development being created on the north side.

Walk Description

You will see a lot of "new" Williamsburg on this walk, but start with a piece of the old. Cross Metropolitan Avenue to Macri Triangle, a little park tucked beneath the highway. At the corner with Union Avenue is a World War II memorial. The surnames listed, along with the bocce court behind the monument, reveal the neighborhood's former character. Italians started settling in Williamsburg for the factory work in the late 19th century, and some old-school Italian bakeries, butcher shops, and social clubs remain between here and Graham Avenue—which is conamed Via Vespucci—to the east.

Walk on Metropolitan with the park on your right. Under the highway, fork right onto North 6th Street.

Turn left on Havemeyer Street. A group of Romanesque buildings on this block were all once affiliated with the Church of the Annunciation. The first one you reach on your right was a convent, converted to apartments in the 1980s but still bearing a cross at the top. The school next to it at #70 was built around the same time. See the Latin inscription at the North 5th Street corner, then cross over to the triangle opposite the church. This offers an excellent vantage point for the school's belfry as well as the church itself (1869) and the rectory to the right of it. Annunciation parish was founded by Germans in 1863, but the church has had a Lithuanian congregation since 1914. If you can, take a look at its ornate interior.

Cross Metropolitan Avenue and go to the right. Visit the ❶ City Reliquary at #370. This unique museum presents the history, culture, and geology of New York City through small objects—anything from seltzer bottles, Statue of Liberty souvenirs, and subway tokens to rock and soil samples, retail signage, and architectural fragments. Across the street is the Knitting Factory, an icon of Manhattan's downtown music scene that relocated to Williamsburg in 2009 and now stands amid a cluster of popular nightspots and restaurants. Look up from street level at the attractive building to your left at Havemeyer. Next to it on Metropolitan, you might mistake Fette Sau for the body shop it *used* to be, but it's one of the city's most highly rated barbecue restaurants.

Turn left at Roebling Street, where graffiti and dramatic fire stairs highlight the side of a terrific old factory building.

Make a right on Fillmore Place, a landmarked block. A pair of real estate investors built 24 rowhouses here in the mid-1850s—20 of them survive, making this the rare pre–Civil War development that's still (mostly) intact. All the homes on your left with stoops and on your right through #13 were erected between 1853 and 1855, during the brief period when Williamsburgh—then spelled with an *h* at the end—was an independent city. These were called "flats buildings" and were meant for the working class, but architecturally they were less like tenements and more like single-family rowhouses built for the well-to-do. For one thing, every room had natural light, as there was just one apartment per floor. Novelist and Williamsburg native Henry Miller wrote in *Tropic of Capricorn* that Fillmore Place was "the most enchanting street I have ever seen."

At Driggs Avenue look across to your right at the flats building (between two empty lots) where Miller lived till the age of 9. But turn left on Driggs. The three buildings to your right were included, along with Miller's former home, in the historic-district designation; they date from the 1860s.

Go right on North 1st Street to Bedford Avenue, ground zero of the hipster-fication of Williamsburg. At the left corner is one of the first places to throw down the artisanal-food gauntlet, Bedford Cheese Shop, which began in a smaller location down the block in 2003 and has spawned a Manhattan outpost.

Turn right on Bedford. Near the next corner, the recreation center on your right was built as a public bathhouse at a time when the area's many tenement dwellers didn't have bathing facilities in their homes. Architect Henry Bacon designed this building the same year his most famous work, the Lincoln Memorial, was completed. Continuing north on Bedford, past North 4th Street on your left, Spoonbill & Sugartown Booksellers is one of the retailers in the former Realform Girdle factory, an early industrial conversion.

Turn right on North 6th Street. To your right at #168 is Figureworks, a gallery dedicated to "art that explores the human form." Farther down on the left, the Spire Lofts is the new residential branding of the property formerly known as St. Vincent de Paul.

Make a left on Driggs. Aside from all the flashy new residences, Williamsburg's older housing stock entails plenty of ordinary flats buildings as well as more-elegant ones, like that on the far left corner of North 7th.

Turn right on North 8th Street. The ❷ **Brooklyn Winery** at #213 gets grapes from upstate and the West Coast, but all production is done on these premises, and you can tour the factory. Or just belly up to the bar and have a taste.

Turn left at Havemeyer. Our Lady of Mount Carmel is the church that sponsors the annual Feast of the Giglio, during which hundreds of men carry a 65-foot, *4-ton* statue of a saint through the streets, accompanied by a brass band that's *on* the structure they're carrying. The summer festival, started by southern Italian immigrants, has been held since 1903—and the *paranza* (lifter) positions are passed down through families.

Go right onto Withers Street, but don't miss the mural that takes up the whole side of the building at Havemeyer and North 9th.

Make a left on Union Avenue and a right on Frost Street. In the ❸ **Brooklyn Art Library** toward the end of the block on your right, you can spend some time thumbing through note-books filled with writing, artwork, doodles, or puzzles by people around the world. The extensive collection comes from the ongoing crowd-sourced Sketchbook Project. A librarian will bring you a few books that match your search criteria, which could be the book's subject, medium, place of origin, or any other category. You can even get started creating your own.

Turn left on Lorimer Street. Watch on your left for the vintage Coca-Cola signs outside Pete's Candy Store, the earliest live-music venue in "new" Williamsburg. When the bar opened in 1999, it simply kept the name of the building's previous occupant. All its shows are still free, and such performers as Norah Jones, Duncan Sheik, Regina Spektor, Joanna Newsom, and Rufus Wain-wright have taken the stage, both pre- and post-fame.

Turn left on Richardson Street. Once you reach the parking lot on your right, you should be able to see a Quonset hut beyond its far corner. This is the clubhouse of the St. Cono American Society, and it contains a shrine to Cono, a saint who hailed from the same town in Italy as the immigrants who established the society in the 1930s. Their social hall sits in the backyard of a member's home—but it's also now behind the luxury high-rises on Bayard Street, offering a juxtaposition of the past and present populaces.

Turn and head in the other direction on Richardson, taking note of the St. Cono honorary street name as you cross Lorimer. In the midst of myriad new buildings, a 1920s classic stands on the right, with busts at the fourth-floor windows and decorative embossed panels. Toward the end on your left, the ❹ **New York Distilling Company** produces gin and rye whiskey, which you can enjoy in a craft cocktail at the in-house bar, the Shanty.

Turn left on Leonard Street. Cross Bayard Street and go only as far as you need to see the ❺ **McCarren Park** pool. The largest (capacity: 6,800) of 11 public swimming pools constructed in New York City by the WPA during the Depression, it had been closed for 20 years and was an overgrown mess when hipsters started using it for concerts and parties, which lead to its refur-bishment and reopening for swimming in 2012.

Return to Bayard and walk alongside the park. This street was completely transformed within a decade—it's mostly new luxury apartment buildings end to end, with a new museum sand-wiched in: MOFAD Lab, run by the ❻ **Museum of Food and Drink.** Celebrating an aspect of our culture that the Smithsonian hasn't gotten around to, the museum holds exhibits, seminars, tastings, and cooking demonstrations.

The homes to your left down Lorimer provide quite a contrast with the bigger, fancier residences lining Bayard. But go to your right at Lorimer to see the bathhouse and pool entrance, all part of the landmarked and renovated recreation complex.

Continue on Lorimer and go into the park on your left, then follow the path to the right. The Tom Stofka Garden on your right is a tranquil, shady spot to take a break. Then resume walking on the path that encircles the running track. About midway down on the other side, exit on your right and cross Union Avenue into another pocket of the park, with a dog run on your right and community garden to your left. Walk through it toward the onion domes of the Russian Orthodox Cathedral of the Transfiguration of Our Lord, which was built from 1916 to 1921 and purportedly modeled after the czar's Winter Palace in St. Petersburg.

Facing the church, go to the right on North 12th. If you wish to avoid the free-admission crowd at the pool in McCarren Park, you can fork over 60 bucks or more for a day pass to the outdoor pool atop the McCarren Hotel, situated opposite the park past Bedford Avenue. The hotel also has a rooftop bar (with daily happy hour) open year-round.

Make a left on Berry Street. Just a few steps away from the McCarren-bordering nouveau architecture, you're surrounded here by the traditional edifices of Williamsburg—built for factories and warehouses, though many have been repurposed.

Turn right on North 11th Street. The large building midblock on your left was constructed in 1896 for the factory, offices, and showroom of Hecla Iron Works, which created all 133 original kiosks of the IRT subway (today's numbered lines) and contributed architectural and ornamental metalwork to other significant structures around the city. This cast-iron facade, manufactured by Hecla itself, demonstrates the company's foresight: it is much thinner than what was typical at the time (think Soho) and eschewed those chunky columns, thus serving as a sort of prototype of the "curtain wall" facade that would become standard several decades later. Another interesting aspect of the design: the central four-pane section of each window pivots open.

Farther along on your right is the taproom of the **7** **Brooklyn Brewery,** which in 1996 returned an industry to Brooklyn that once accounted for 1 in 10 beers drunk in the United States but had died with the closing of the Schaefer and Rheingold breweries in the mid-1970s. Brooklyn Brewery led the way for the city's numerous craft breweries that would open in the 2000s and has become a worldwide ambassador for the borough.

At Wythe Avenue, the hotel so brashly proclaimed at the corner is the Wythe, a boutique property with an art curator on staff. Go into the lobby to see the latest exhibit—and maybe head up to the über-trendy rooftop bar for drinks with a view. The Wythe's building was erected in 1901 for a wooden-cask plant. Turn left on Wythe Avenue, and behold another new industrial-chic hotel on your right at North 10th. Here, you look *down* at a bar—sunken from the sidewalk. There's also one inside a watertower on the roof. Facing the Williamsburg, you can see yet another new hotel down Wythe to your right. That's the William Vale, with commercial space in its triangular-girded bottom and 183 guest rooms—every one of them with a balcony—in the upper half. It also has a rooftop bar, as well as an elevated public park.

Turn right onto North 10th, then left on Kent Avenue. Bushwick Inlet Park is being expanded up to North 12th Street (where the inlet is actually located), but for now enter at North 9th and go to the right. You can climb a zigzagging path up the grassy "bleachers" and plop down to watch the Manhattan skyline or a soccer game. Then head south into adjacent ❽ **East River State Park,** past rail-track and cement pillar remnants from the shipping terminal that was in operation here from the 1870s to 1983. Read about its history on signs near the North 8th Street entrance.

Follow the cobblestone path toward the water. It turns gravelly before reaching a sandy beach. Relax as you see fit here, then head back toward the North 8th gate, noting the cement floors and wall foundations of the demolished terminal warehouses to your right. The Smorgasburg food bazaar is held here on Saturdays in season. Make a right on Kent.

Turn right on North 7th Street, then swoop along the street between the Edge North condo (#34) and Level (formerly known as the Edge III). Make a right at North 6th Street in front of #22, the Edge South. Proceed along the waterfront esplanade and onto the stylishly designed North 5th Street pier. Wend your way one block farther, and return to Kent Avenue via North 4th Street, passing 1 North 4th and the Northside Piers complex on your left. None of these towers—containing nearly 2,000 apartments total—existed before 2008; the area wasn't even zoned for residential until 2005.

The massive six-story Austin Nichols building on your right *was* here prior to 2008—almost a hundred years prior, in fact. Its architect was Cass Gilbert, who designed the Woolworth Building around the same time. By the time this former warehouse was considered for landmark status in 2005, it was tattered and unremarkable-looking. The landmarks commission voted in favor of it nonetheless, but that designation was overturned by the city council. So Mayor Michael Bloomberg vetoed the revocation by the council . . . which then overruled his veto. Unlandmarked, the building was rehabbed and converted to apartments by a developer who donated a deed of easement in exchange for a tax break. That easement permanently prohibits the addition of any stories—which was a main concern of the pro-landmarking faction in the first place. For earlier history about the building, read the plaque next to the door.

Turn right on Kent. Let loose at OddFellows Ice Cream parlor on your left. Flavors might include black pepper fig, miso cherry, cornbread, and PB&J. Don't worry; they make vanilla, too! Is it cruel that SoulCycle opened across the street? Continuing down Kent, you can still find reminders that this whole area was a virtual ghost town when we entered the 21st century. Some old commercial buildings await the wrecking ball, others just sit there with a yet-to-be-determined fate. When you've crossed North 1st Street, turn and look back at a vista of glassy high-rises foregrounded by graffiti-covered old warehouses—at least for the time being.

One block farther, at Grand Street, you can see ahead to the chimney and surrounding buildings of the old Domino Sugar refinery, which closed down in 2004 after more than 150 years on the Williamsburg waterfront. The mural on Grand tells about life in "Los Sures," the traditionally Latino south side of Williamsburg, with an emphasis on Domino's importance to the community. Check out one last thing before you turn on Grand: a building diagonally across the intersection from the mural—the second one in from Kent, with four tall arches across the front. It was built in 1889 for the North Side Bank, its location chosen because of all the potential customers coming and going from the ferry at the foot of Grand Street.

Walk on Grand toward the river. ㊹ **Grand Ferry Park** was the *only* patch of Williamsburg waterfront accessible to the public before 2007. Read the history of the site on the smokestack left behind by Pfizer; if you're wondering why the pharmaceutical giant was mixing molasses here, it contributed to penicillin production.

Buses on Kent or Wythe will drop you at a subway, or go back to North 6th for the East River ferry. If you choose to walk the 10 blocks to the L at Bedford and North 7th, take Wythe or Berry—those avenues and the streets off them are full of restaurants, taverns, coffee bars, and other dining and drinking destinations, including Mast Brothers chocolate factory and shop, Brooklyn Oenology's tasting room, and the Radegast beer garden, plus performance venues such as National Sawdust and the Music Hall of Williamsburg. You can also return to Manhattan via the Williamsburg Bridge: head up Grand, make a right on Bedford Avenue, and access the bridge via a ramp between South 5th and South 6th. Visit El Museo de Los Sures at 120 South 1st St., off Bedford, en route.

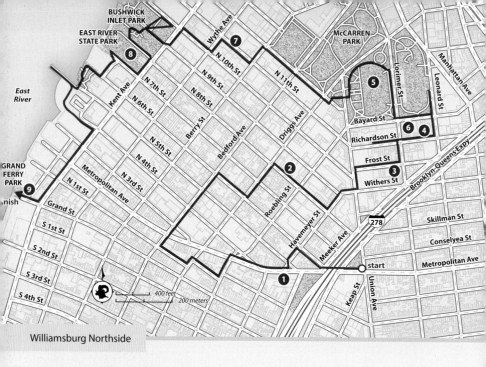

Williamsburg Northside

Points of Interest

1. **City Reliquary** 370 Metropolitan Ave.; 718-782-4842, cityreliquary.org
2. **Brooklyn Winery** 213 N. 8th St.; 347-763-1506, bkwinery.com
3. **Brooklyn Art Library** 28 Frost St.; 718 302-3770, sketchbookproject.com/library
4. **New York Distilling Company** 79 Richardson St.; 718-412-0874, nydistilling.com
5. **McCarren Park** Bayard Street and Lorimer Street; nycgovparks.org
6. **Museum of Food and Drink (MOFAD) Lab** 62 Bayard St.; 718-387-2845, mofad.org
7. **Brooklyn Brewery** 79 N. 11th St.; 718-486-7422, brooklynbrewery.com
8. **East River State Park** Kent Avenue and North 8th Street; 718-782-2731, parks.ny.gov/parks/155/details.aspx
9. **Grand Ferry Park** Grand Street west of Kent Avenue; nycgovparks.org

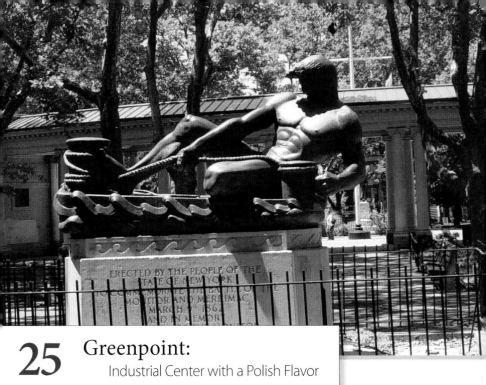

25 Greenpoint:
Industrial Center with a Polish Flavor

Above: A monument in Monsignor McGolrick Park honors the legendary but doomed warship Monitor, *which was built in Greenpoint*

BOUNDARIES: India St., Monitor St., Driggs Ave., East River
DISTANCE: 4.3 miles
SUBWAY: G to Nassau Ave.

Greenpoint's factories used to churn out so much smoke, its major industries were dubbed the "black arts." In the late 19th century, more than 50 oil refineries and 20 glass factories were in operation, and those smoke-spewing industries also included printing, ironworking, and porcelain manufacturing. They were all on the decline by the mid–20th century, but today Greenpoint is a production center of a different kind. Light manufacturing and a whole range of designers and creative entities now populate rehabbed and subdivided old industrial structures, while culinary artisans have filled many storefronts. For over a century, however, Greenpoint's most steadfast identity has been as the Polish capital of New York City. Poles first arrived in the huge wave of Eastern European immigration of the late 1800s, and the influx didn't abate as later generations fled Nazism, then communism, then postcommunist uncertainty.

Walk Description

Walk west on Nassau Avenue, going straight onto Bedford Avenue at Lorimer Street (where Nassau and Bedford cross). Enter ❶ **Father Jerzy Popieluszko Square** to your right. The murdered anticommunist priest is honored with a granite bust and a garden of colorful flowers. Be sure to find the smaller sculpture of outstretched arms—symbolizing the yearning for freedom and peace—on the other side of the flagpole in the square; it can get obscured by foliage.

Leave the small park on the other side, which returns you to Nassau Avenue, and go to the left. A block and a half along on your right, the Lot has created a hipster paradise replete with hammock, pink flamingos, and a repurposed shipping container from where the Lot radio streams music online and over speakers.

Continue one more block on Nassau, then go to your left, walking between the high school and the tennis courts. Cross Bedford and enter McCarren Park, a 35-acre green space that sprawls across five blocks and demarcates Greenpoint from Williamsburg (both neighborhoods claim the park; see more on Walk 24). Follow the path to your left, then curve right as you pass the comfort station. Bypass the corner park gate, exiting in the middle of the block on Lorimer Street, opposite a garage, and go to the right.

Turn left on Driggs Avenue. The diamond-patterned apartment house on your left after crossing Leonard Street has the statue of an eagle—a national symbol of Poland—at the top. Down the block to your right, the Polish National Home (est. 1914) is a cultural and social-services center that keeps the homeland's heritage alive for immigrants and their American-born children; it houses a popular nightspot named Warsaw. Take a look at the historical murals to your right at Eckford Street, then continue on Driggs. You'll come to Father Studzinski Square, a not always well-maintained patch between Graham Avenue and McGuinness Boulevard that honors a longtime pastor of Greenpoint's major Polish church, St. Stanislaus, which you encounter two blocks farther along. Affectionately called St. Stans, the commanding church has stood here since the 1890s. Street signs outside it commemorate visits by Lech Walesa and Pope John Paul II. Its marble interior is worth seeing.

Go one more block on Driggs and enter ❷ **Monsignor McGolrick Park** at Russell Street. Walk through the allée of trees to the colonnaded shelter, erected in 1910. There's an angel statue in memory of World War I vets on the flagpole side of the pavilion, and a larger monument on the other side in honor of the USS *Monitor*, the Civil War ship that was built at Greenpoint's Continental Iron Works. The first iron-hulled ship deployed by the Navy, the *Monitor* famously battled the *Merrimack* at Hampton Roads, Virginia. (A *Monitor* museum is supposed to open someday on the Greenpoint waterfront.)

Go back through the shelter pavilion and walk in the direction the angel is facing. Leave the park between gates crowned with munching-squirrel statuettes and head to your right on Russell Street.

Make a left on Nassau. Polish businesses are interspersed with trendier arrivals like a ramen shop and coffeehouse. Pop into a Polish bakery if you have a hankering for babka or a big jelly doughnut.

Turn right on McGuinness Boulevard. To your right, the Polish & Slavic Federal Credit Union's facade depicts coats of arms of various cities in Poland—the mermaid, for instance, is a symbol of Warsaw. Also see its mural of Polish heroes in the adjacent parking lot.

Turn left on Norman Avenue, where Brooklyn's oldest public elementary school stands. A mere decade or so before P.S. 34 was built in 1867, Greenpoint had been a rural community where children were still educated privately—but then the population soared with the growth of the shipbuilding industry.

Turn right on Manhattan Avenue, the neighborhood's main commercial thoroughfare. Two eras are represented at #723: the store owes its classically styled facade to the building's original existence as a 1920s theater, while the ramp, oval floor, and disco ball(!) inside remain from its later incarnation as a roller rink. Go check them out, and also look at the ceiling ornamentation. Meanwhile, the cast-iron "bishop's crook" street lamps along the avenue and the turn-of-the-century sidewalk clock in front of #733 hark back to a more distant age. Look up at #735 and enjoy those terra cotta faces in the window panels. Continue on Manhattan to Calyer Street, where the left corner reminds us of the days when people didn't just dash in and out of the ATM vestibule, so a bank would build a majestic structure like this 1908 Pantheon simulacrum with a stunning marble interior.

Turn left on Calyer. As you cross Lorimer, take note of those original iron banisters and fences in front of the 1880s brick rowhouses to your right—and of iron accents on residences throughout the neighborhood. They're a source of hometown pride, given Greenpoint's ironworking heritage. Past Lorimer to your right are three frame houses from 1868 that have all been re-sided, to varying aesthetic effect. The first one was built for a member of the Calyer family.

Make a right on Guernsey. On this side of the Calyer-facing house to your right, a cast-iron pillar stands beside the window. It's a relic from the storefront that originally occupied the circa-1870 building's ground floor. Head the short distance down Guernsey to the three brick residences facing you on Oak Street. The large one in the corner, set back behind a front lawn, was built in 1887 as the Greenpoint Home for the Aged. The architect was Theobald Engelhardt, who designed many homes, churches, and factories in Greenpoint, Williamsburg, and Bushwick, often hired by fellow German-American businessmen.

Return to Calyer and go right. Then make your first left. When and why this one block—the tail end of a street named Dobbin—was renamed Clifford Place is unknown. The houses to see here are the cute circa-1880 quintet on your left with the boxy window bays that have been refaced in different types of shingles.

Go back to Calyer and continue in the direction you'd been going. The road bends on its way west, with ❸ **Triskelion Arts** capping the block on your left. Triskelion specializes in dance but also presents comedy and clown shows, film festivals, and plays.

Turn right on Franklin Street, which has developed into a shopping destination for vintage clothing and furnishings.

Make a right on Noble Street, where #93, 95, 101, 103, 105, and 107 were all built between 1851 and 1854, among the oldest houses in the neighborhood. On your left at #108 is Greenpoint's sole remaining synagogue, Ahawath Israel (1904), which closed for a while but has been revitalized by newcomers. Toward the end on your left, Union Baptist Church, built in 1863, *has* been vacated. But a still-vital institution dwells next door: the Polish National Alliance, or Zjednoczenie Polsko Narodowe—see the ZPN imprinted in the stoop—a longstanding fraternal and social-services organization. Also see the "grotesques" peering down from the roof.

Turn left on Manhattan Avenue. Go into ❹ **Sunshine Laundromat** at #820. It doesn't matter that you don't have laundry to do—walk past the washing machines and through a door at the rear made out of dryer doors. Sunshine was the first laundromat ever issued a liquor license, and now you know why. . . .

Two doors away, but visible up and down the avenue, is the church that has given Greenpoint a skyline since 1873, and one that's considered the Brooklyn masterpiece of architect Patrick Keely, who designed about 600 Catholic churches nationwide. Many of his churches served Irish-immigrant congregations, as St. Anthony originally did. It later merged with St. Alphonsus, a German church, though today the parishioners are primarily Polish or Latino.

Opposite the church, that's not an Alpine ski lodge but a recently restored 1887 commercial building dubbed Keramos Hall—after the locally produced Keramos vase, which itself was named after the Longfellow poem "Kéramos," about a potter. The vase was made by Greenpoint-based Union Porcelain Works, whose owner Thomas C. Smith developed this building with stores, professional offices, and meeting rooms for civic organizations under its roof. Union Porcelain tiles are between the steps of the doorway beneath the tower. Also look for delicate woodworking in and around the recessed upper wing to the right.

Make a left on Milton, an elegant street, due largely to Smith, who launched Union Porcelain after a 30-plus-year career as an architect and became a major real estate developer in Greenpoint as well. He designed the first two houses on your left, an attached pair of 1868 Second Empires. His own residence was the 1867 mini-mansion at #136 that's now a Reformed church. Smith's Union Porcelain was the first US maker of what had previously been an exclusively European product, and several leading museums, including the Metropolitan and the Brooklyn Museum, hold its pieces in their collections.

To your right, St. John's Lutheran Church was designed by prolific Theobald Engelhardt for a parish of German immigrants—as indicated by the church's name above the door. Engelhardt also designed the lovely Queen Anne duo (1889) at #124 and 122. Smith is responsible for the three houses that follow, which are entered on the side. Across the street, all the houses set back from the sidewalk were developed by Smith.

You will proceed west on Milton, but at Franklin, pause to browse in ❺ WORD at the left corner. A de facto community center, the bookstore holds events every night during some weeks and has a wide range of themed reading groups. When WORD opened in 2007, Franklin was a somewhat neglected street, but it has since been revived with a slew of boutiques, bars, and bistros. Located just one block from the waterfront factories, Franklin had been Greenpoint's busiest commercial street in the 1800s—that's why the earliest houses on Milton and Noble are near this end.

Turn left from Milton onto West Street and enter Greenpoint Terminal at #61–67, one of the few structures to survive a suspicious 10-alarm fire in 2006 that gutted most of the four-block-long Greenpoint Terminal Market—built for the American Manufacturing Co., once the world's largest rope maker, with a Brooklyn workforce of more than 2,000 in the 1910s. The cool interior architecture entails sky bridges, staircases, metal beams, and more. Artists and designers have galleries, studios, and showrooms in the building, so drop in on whichever interest you. When you've finished exploring inside, go out to West and turn left. Go left down the alley opposite Milton, all the way to the water, for the Brooklyn Barge, where you can climb aboard a historic vessel or just imbibe at the floating bar.

Back on West, go one more block to Greenpoint Avenue, turn left, and keep walking until you're in ❻ WNYC Transmitter Park. Enjoy its pier, pedestrian bridge traversing a defunct ferry slip, and *fab-u-lous* views. As you might have guessed, this is the former site of the public-radio station's transmission towers—and if all goes according to plan, the esplanade will eventually be extended along the entire shoreline. Sit, recline, or roam as much as you'd like here, then exit near the 1930s transmission house onto Kent Street and make a right.

Turn right on West Street. The buildings to your left, dating to around 1870, were all part of the complex where a math teacher's best friend, the Eberhard Faber pencil, was manufactured from 1872 until the company relocated to Pennsylvania in 1956. Turn left on Greenpoint Avenue for their main building—sharpened pencils are part of its facade, as is the star-in-diamond trademark of Eberhard Faber's Mongol pencils. Across the street, among the restaurants that have opened in this rejuvenated "pencil factory district," is Paulie Gee's, cited in many best-pizza-in-NYC rankings.

Continue on Greenpoint Avenue. To your left across Franklin is the impressive terra cotta–adorned side of an 1895 bank building that has housed the Polish Home Service and offices of the Polish daily newspaper *Nowy Dziennik*.

Make a left on Manhattan, then a left on Kent—another lovely residential block with various home styles represented. The charming church on your right was built in 1870 and vacated by its last congregation around 2007. The wing on the right with an angled window was originally the Sunday school, and we're not sure why the teeny passage (with round window) that connects it to the church needed a door, but it's cute. By this point you might be able to recognize the house next to it (#143) as the work of Theobald Engelhardt.

Now meet another influential figure in Greenpoint history: steamship builder Neziah Bliss, who was one of the first industrialists to set up shop here and who had some of the early roads built. He lived in #130, his daughter and son-in-law in #132; they were both constructed for Bliss in 1859. Midway down on the right is Greenpoint's oldest house of worship in continuous use, Church of the Ascension, built in 1865 for an Episcopal congregation.

Turn right at Franklin. The full block on your right from Java to India Street is occupied by the Astral, erected in 1886 for employees of Charles Pratt's Astral Oil. It was an upgrade from the dreadful flats most working-class people were crowded into at the time and, unlike those typical tenements, it had natural light, indoor plumbing, hot water—and magnificent exteriors.

Turn right on India Street. Farther down, the apartment house at #104 is where Hannah lived on HBO's *Girls*. Back at Manhattan Avenue is an entrance to the G train.

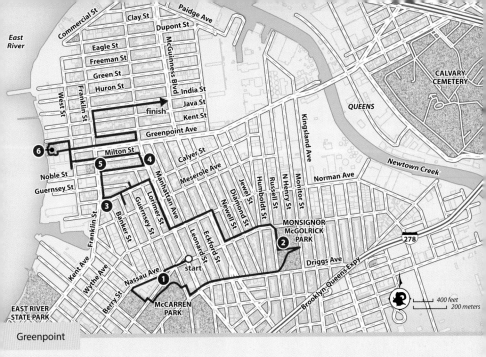

Points of Interest

1. **Father Jerzy Popieluszko Square** Lorimer Street between Nassau and Bedford Avenues; nycgovparks.org

2. **Monsignor McGolrick Park** Driggs Avenue and Russell Street; nycgovparks.org

3. **Triskelion Arts** 106 Calyer St., 718-389-3473, triskelionarts.org

4. **Sunshine Laundromat** 860 Manhattan Ave.; 718-475-2055, facebook.com/pg/sunshine.pinball

5. **WORD** 126 Franklin St.; 718-383-0096, wordbookstores.com

6. **WNYC Transmitter Park** Kent Street to Greenpoint Avenue west of West Street; nycgovparks.org

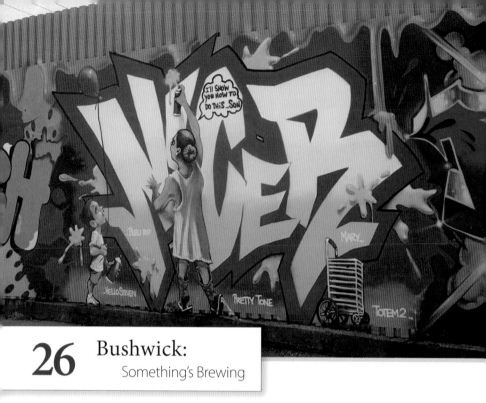

26 Bushwick:
Something's Brewing

Above: Streets like Troutman are an outdoor gallery of murals, curated by the Bushwick Collective

BOUNDARIES: Cypress Ave., Linden St., Broadway, Ellery St.
DISTANCE: 4.6 miles
SUBWAY: L to Jefferson St. (exit SE corner of Starr and Wyckoff)

Not so long ago, the idea of people flocking to Bushwick for an evening out or paying $2,500 a month for a studio apartment there was unfathomable. After all, we could still remember that night in July 1977 when looters and arsonists nearly destroyed Bushwick during a citywide black-out. Bushwick was plagued by crime and poverty throughout the late decades of the 20th century, and while community social-services initiatives and low-income housing improvements set it on an upswing in the 1990s, it remained one of the city's poorest districts. But then came the hipsters—first because they were getting priced out of Williamsburg but soon because Bushwick was developing an artsy, adventurous culture and lifestyle all its own. Now Bushwick has arrived, and it is producing the newest wave in creativity and dining. You'll see some of it on the first leg of this walk, before you trek through an industrial area to reach the most historic part of this large neighborhood.

Walk Description

At the top of the subway stairs, do a 180 and walk west on Wyckoff Avenue, commencing your tour of Bushwick's street art. On your left at Jefferson Street, that giant YES on a former warehouse marks the House of Yes, which despite the conspicuous sign is considered an underground arts venue. All-night dance parties are among the events held here, but their specialty is aerial circus performance, often with a burlesque edge. Turn right on Jefferson, right on Scott Avenue, and left on Troutman Street to view additional murals.

The art loop continues with a right on Cypress Avenue, right on Starr Street, right on St. Nicholas Avenue, and left on Troutman. Across Wyckoff on your right, ❶ **Kings County Brewers Collective** got Bushwick back in the beer-making business upon its opening in 2016. (In the years before Prohibition, Bushwick was home to 14 breweries.) Run by three guys who met at a home-brewers club, KCBC has production facilities in back and a bar up front.

Turn left on Irving, then right on Starr, walking alongside Maria Hernandez Park, the recreational hub of the community. Its name is a reminder of Bushwick's troubled past. Hernandez was a community activist who tried to rid the streets of drugs but was shot to death in 1989 by dealers who fired into the window of her apartment (on the next block of Starr).

Turn right on Knickerbocker Avenue. Prior to 2010, this stretch was full of mom-and-pop Hispanic businesses. Now it has trendy restaurants and shops where you can buy $35-a-pound cheese. It starts to get more industrial past Melrose Street.

Cross Flushing Avenue and drop in on the ground floor of the former pillow factory to your right for the ❷ **Shops at the Loom,** a so-called hipster mini-mall of boutiques plus a coffee bar and cobblestoned courtyard. Workspace on the upper levels is dedicated to creative industries.

Back on Knickerbocker, proceed in the direction you'd been heading into another major street-art zone. This is also a center of the dining and nightlife scene in Bushwick.

Turn left on Grattan Street. So many popular places are concentrated in the area, the name Morgantown was coined for it. Pop into any of them and you'll probably feel like you're in the coolest backyard or living room ever. One mainstay is on your left after Morgan Avenue: Pine Box Rock Shop, a vegan bar (yes, that applies to booze) and performance venue. "Pine Box" refers to the building's previous use—casket manufacturing.

Turn right at Bogart Street, beneath the BogArt, which helped put Bushwick on the cultural radar. This ex-factory contains studios upstairs, art galleries at street and basement levels.

From Bogart, go onto Seigel Street. The first door on the left is ❸ **Fine & Raw Chocolate** factory, whose stated mission is "to save the world through silliness and chocolate." The eco-friendly operation not only uses organic, free-trade cacao beans to make chocolate bars, truffles, and spreads, but the wrappers are made from recycled paper and labeled in vegetable-based ink.

Head back to Bogart and make a right. Then go right on Moore Street to the famous red door on the right. Here's the restaurant that launched Bushwick to the foodie forefront, Roberta's—purveyor of much-ballyhooed pizzas and also of the local culinary aesthetic, one that involves ingredients growing on site, some type of art or media (in this case, an epicurean internet radio show) being produced along with the food, and an overall DIY postindustrial vibe. As if the pizza accolades weren't enough, Roberta's has opened a bakery on the other side of its patio.

Stay on Moore, then turn left on White Street. Go left at Cook Street, the first of several consecutive quick turns. Follow it with a right on Evergreen Avenue and left on Flushing Avenue.

Turn right on Central Avenue, and enter ❹ **Green Central Knoll** on your right. It has a streambed, which may or may not have water flowing. Not that it matters, as the fish are made of metal. The name Green Central Knoll may sound like a topographical description, but it's actually a compendium of the streets bordering the park: (Ever)green, Central, and Noll. Follow the "stream" and then keep going to exit the park on Evergreen Avenue, where you make a right.

Turn left on Flushing Avenue. A residential village is due to take shape on your left.

Turn left on Bushwick Avenue. Another apartment building is going up to your left at Montieth Street. All this land being redeveloped used to be owned by Rheingold, which was the last Bushwick brewery to close, in 1976. Green Central Knoll was the eastern end of Rheingold's 7-acre spread. When you reach Forrest Street, the homes to your left, right, and ahead of you are Renaissance Estates and Rheingold Gardens, a complex of two-family houses, condominiums, and rental apartments that was built on part of Rheingold's site in the early 2000s.

Turn right on Garden Street, and down the block go left onto the walkway through the playground. Follow it to Beaver Street, then cross over and walk on Ellery Street. There's a majestic school on the left, built in 1883, which has been turned into an artists' residence and collective—they occasionally present exhibitions and indie-rock shows.

Make a left on Broadway. Check out the lovely building at #822, a reminder that this was once a more elegant street. Broadway in Bushwick suffered the worst devastation of any place in the entire city during the 1977 blackout. Most store owners lived outside the neighborhood, and they'd already gone home when the lights went out at 9:30 p.m. The police force had been drastically reduced due to NYC's financial crisis, so looters took over, tearing off security gates and stealing hoards of merchandise. Forty-five Broadway stores were burned down, and nearly a hundred others damaged. Broadway's vacancy rate soared past 40 percent after the blackout.

Turn left on Locust Street. Toward the end of the block on the right is the old Ulmer Brewery's storehouse and stable, built in 1890. Make a right on Beaver Street for the main Ulmer building where the "lagerbier" was actually brewed. The white plaque with the company's name is on the original brewery, which was enlarged with the buildings to the right around 1881. Turn right at Belvidere Street. The highlight of this landmarked site is Ulmer's charming 1885 office. A *U* is embossed prominently at the top and on the left and right edges of the building.

Turn left on Broadway. Then make a left at Arion Place, and as you're doing so, look up to your right for the WALL ST. etched on the corner building. This building was designed in 1884 by architect Theobald Engelhardt for his own offices. He designed the Ulmer brewery and many other Bushwick structures. The street's name would be changed owing to another Engelhardt project, that arch-windowed redbrick building on your left. This was built, believe it or not, for a glee club, Arion Männerchor. It stamped its musicality on the front, with lyre designs in the balcony railings and corners of the roof (Arion is a lyre player in Greek mythology). Such singing societies thrived in German-immigrant neighborhoods like Bushwick, but this was an especially successful one. It had its own orchestra and even toured Germany and performed at the White House for President Theodore Roosevelt. In addition to the top-floor concert hall, the 1887 building contained a ballroom, wine cellar, bowling alleys, and a billiards room. In 2003 it was converted to apartments under the name Opera House Lofts.

Turn right on Bushwick Avenue. Midblock past Melrose Street, #603 is ❺ **Silent Barn,** a multi-disciplinary artists' collective—or "experimental sandbox," as it's described—with apartments for artists as well as shared work studios. It also holds public performances, readings, and exhibitions.

On the next block on your right, the exteriors of St. Mark's Evangelical Lutheran church and school are being preserved in the site's conversion to apartments, so you should still be able to read the German inscription at the base of the pillar near Jefferson Street. Both buildings were designed by Theobald Engelhardt and dedicated in 1892.

Walk beneath the train at Myrtle Avenue and commence your stroll along the Boulevard, as Bushwick Avenue was known in its highfalutin days when beer barons had their mansions here. That one on your right with the conical tower was designed by Engelhardt in 1889 for the owner of the local Claus Lipsius Brewery, but is more often identified with a subsequent owner, Dr. Frederick Cook, who had the juicier life story. Cook, the son of German immigrants, was on the medical team that accompanied Robert Peary's Arctic expeditions in the 1890s and also was an explorer in his own right. His claim of reaching the North Pole in April 1908—one year before Peary—could not be substantiated, and the ensuing investigation also discredited his earlier claim of being the first American to summit Mount McKinley. Cook later served seven years in jail for stock fraud, but was eventually pardoned by President Franklin D. Roosevelt. Be sure to take a few steps down Willoughby Avenue so you can see the house from all angles. Do the same across Bushwick Avenue at the *Victory With Peace* statue.

The row of five townhouses across Willoughby from the war memorial were built in the late 1880s for William Ulmer, whose brewery you saw earlier. The homes—also the work of Engelhardt—were most likely employee housing, though given their fine style (pardon the alterations), they would have been for managers rather than line workers. The two apartment houses at the end of the block on your left and the (variously modified) wood-frame houses with porches across Suydam Street to your right are additional Engelhardt designs for the middle class.

Continuing on Bushwick, you'll notice the profile of Victorian mansions amid rowhouses in different styles and states of repair. The Classical Revival library on your right at DeKalb Avenue was built in 1905 through the endowment of Andrew Carnegie that gave Brooklyn 20 of its library branches. The school opposite it was constructed in the 1870s for a "Home for the Aged" that was run by the Little Sisters of the Poor and remained open until 1970.

Another two blocks brings you to ❻ **South Bushwick Reformed Church,** which predates the beer-boom-funded construction of most of old Bushwick Avenue. It's been here since 1853, built for a congregation founded in 1654. Many just call it the White Church, for obvious reasons.

Turn left on Greene Avenue and right on Central Avenue, and proceed to elaborate St. Barbara, a twin-towered Baroque fantasia built on the largesse of local brewer Leonard Eppig, who had a daughter named Barbara. Enjoy the abundantly carved front, then trot down Bleeker Street to examine that side. Return to Central and continue east.

Turn right at Grove Street. Back at Bushwick Avenue, you're between two fine mansions built in 1890 for German businessmen. To your right, don't miss the eyebrow windows and curlicue roof finials. Across the avenue from the turreted mansion on your left is a redbrick mansion built for Louis Bossert, a German-born lumber mogul, in 1887. It later became Arion Männerchor's clubhouse when the singing group could no longer sustain its palatial quarters on Arion Place.

Go left on Bushwick. At the next corner, the house to your left takes Queen Anne quirkiness to new heights—or, more accurately, new girths. Opposite it, check out the terra cotta dragons and wrought-iron roof cresting on the attractive redbricker that's not a mansion but the end house of a Queen Anne row. Turn right on Linden Street to see the face in the triangle at the very top.

Continue down Linden to Broadway. The Gates Ave. J/M/Z station is just to your right.

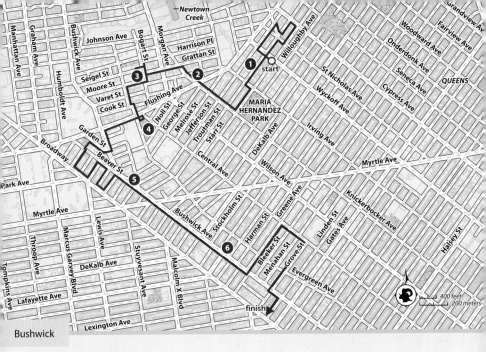

Points of Interest

1 **Kings County Brewers Collective** 381 Troutman St.; kcbcbeer.com

2 **Shops at the Loom** 1087 Flushing Ave.; 718-417-1616, shopsattheloom.com

3 **Fine & Raw Chocolate** 288 Seigel St.; 718-366-3633, fineandraw.com

4 **Green Central Knoll** South of Flushing Avenue between Evergreen and Central Avenues; nycgovparks.org

5 **Silent Barn** 603 Bushwick Ave.; silentbarn.org

6 **South Bushwick Reformed Church** 855 Bushwick Ave.; 347-350-6110, southbushwickchurch.org

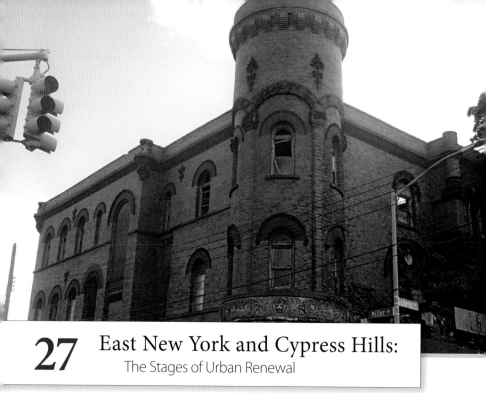

27 East New York and Cypress Hills:
The Stages of Urban Renewal

Above: This castle at Liberty and Miller Avenues was built for the 75th Precinct

BOUNDARIES: Highland Blvd., Linwood St., New Lots Ave., Pennsylvania Ave.
DISTANCE: 4.3 miles
SUBWAY: C to Liberty Ave.

East New York is a large neighborhood extending from the Queens border that runs through Highland Park all the way south to Jamaica Bay. This route is mostly confined to its northwest quadrant, yet the walk is lengthy because it covers two subcommunities: Cypress Hills, considered a separate neighborhood by those who live there, and historic New Lots. Outsiders may only know East New York from its troubled reputation, but many residents have a strong sense of community and deep family roots in the area. Among the hardest hit of NYC neighborhoods by drugs, crime, and poverty from the late 1960s into the '90s, it's a resurgent neighborhood today, and the urban renewal has been driven primarily by church and civic groups.

Walk Description

Exit at the northwest corner of Liberty Avenue and Pennsylvania/Granville Payne Avenue, and step around to the front entrance of a building described by the *Brooklyn Eagle* upon its opening in 1922 as a "handsome, but not extravagant, structure, with all the up-to-date appointments of a first-class bank" (mahogany furnishings among them). It's been used by a religious congregation since the 1970s. Another imposing Classical-style building from the 1920s, also no longer serving its original purpose, stands across Pennsylvania: the former Magistrates Court.

Walk east on Liberty Avenue past the ex-courthouse. Turn right on New Jersey Avenue. This part of East New York was on the German belt that stretched across Brooklyn starting in the second half of the 19th century, and here on your left is a *kirche* for those early German residents, who named it St. Johannes. Built in 1885, it has since converted to ❶ **Grace Baptist.**

Go right on Glenmore Avenue, heading toward the onion domes of Holy Trinity Russian Orthodox Church (1935). Before reaching the church, note the canopies over the doors of #404 and #402. They too have an onion-dome shape—the church installed them after purchasing the houses for the priest, custodian, and choirmaster.

Turn around at Pennsylvania Avenue and retrace your steps on Glenmore, then continue east. The Baptist church past Bradford Street retains indicia of the synagogue for which it was built in 1921. It's one of several converted synagogues in the area, which had a large Jewish population throughout the first half of the 20th century. Danny Kaye, Phil Silvers, Shelley Winters, and John Garfield all grew up in Jewish immigrant families in East New York.

Turn left on Miller Avenue, looking at the back of the ex-synagogue on your way. At the end of the block stands a castle without a dominion. This Romanesque fortress from 1886, constructed for a police precinct station house, has been vacant for a long time, yet you can still enjoy such terrific features as the decorative ironwork and terra cotta lion heads.

Turn left on Liberty Avenue to take in all of the "castle." Turn right on Bradford. Cross Atlantic Avenue, generally considered the boundary between East New York and Cypress Hills. Both communities were absorbed by the town of New Lots when it spun off from Flatbush in the mid-1800s. The black-and-white apartment house on your right was erected in 1873 as New Lots Town Hall.

Make a left on Fulton Street, followed by a right on Wyona Street. On your left you find another late-19th-century church that's altered its identity. It initially served a Reformed congregation founded in 1864. Farther down the street, enter ❷ **George Walker Jr. Park,** offering a wilderness theme in the midst of the city, with sprinklers coming out of faux tree trunks and a path of animal footprints that you should follow to the other end.

Exit the park on Vermont Street and go right.

Turn right at Jamaica Avenue, veering onto Arlington Avenue when they meet past Wyona.

Turn left on Miller Avenue and climb! At the aptly named Highland Boulevard, make a right. Because of the views, this was prime real estate, as you can tell from the lavish homes. On your left after Heath Place, #279 is one of the older ones, constructed in 1900. Another mansion from that year is on the grounds of the Carmelite monastery farther along on your left.

Once you're past the residences, enter ❸ Highland Park at the boulder on your right. Descend the 100-odd steps, and turn left at the bottom. You'll be looking down on tennis courts to your right. Stay to the left when the path splits, but then head downhill to your right between the fields. When the paths diverge toward the bottom, go left, between a playground and baseball diamond, to Linwood Street and Jamaica Avenue.

Turn right on Jamaica Avenue. The house at #494, across from the playground, is from the first half of the 19th century, possibly earlier. As the house was renovated and resold over the years (to people unaware of its history), it had been virtually dropped from the roster of extant Dutch farmhouses, which has dwindled to fewer than a dozen. This Brooklyn section of Highland Park, referred to as the "lower park" (Queens has the "upper park" on the other side of Highland Boulevard), was an addition to the original park, made possible by the city's purchase of the Schencks' farmstead. *Their* colonial-era house remained in the park until the mid–20th century.

Proceeding on Jamaica, watch on your right for the World War I memorial *Dawn of Glory,* a somewhat erotic (for a war monument) statue for which legendary bodybuilder Charles Atlas posed. After Ashford Street, check out the children's garden—first cultivated in 1915. It is the only survivor among the "farm gardens" established in city parks during that social-reform-minded age to provide work, education, and fresh air to tenement-dwelling children. Abandoned in the '70s and '80s, the garden is now tended by both community volunteers and students.

Turn left and go a short block on Warwick Street to Ridgewood Avenue, where you turn left. There's a lot going on at the corner Victorian on your near right at Ashford, what with those various windows and bays; it's calmer and more conventional in front. The house was built in 1904, and Cypress Hills has its fair share of houses from that period, though many have undergone alterations ranging from mild to drastic enough for you to doubt the house's vintage.

Turn right on Linwood. On your right, P.S. 108 is a city landmark and listed on the National Register of Historic Places for its age (built in 1895) and Romanesque styling.

Make a right on Arlington. The block from Cleveland Street to Ashford Street offers a few wraparound porches and pointy turrets. After Ashford, you'll find one of Brooklyn's earliest public libraries. Opened in 1906 to serve the entire "East Branch" of Brooklyn (as the building still says), it's now known as the ④ **Arlington branch.** A corner in the children's room is named for Ezra Jack Keats, the beloved picture-book author, who spent many hours reading in this library when he was growing up in East New York.

At Jerome Street, the house with the mushroom-cap turret on your right was originally owned by a woman who survived the *Titanic*. The lofty brick home diagonally across from it was built for a doctor in 1906.

Keep going on Arlington, a stretch known as Doctors Row. The two houses flanking Barbey Street to your right were constructed at the turn of the century, soon to be followed by #140 on your left. Just a few years after that house was built in 1904, its front door was shifted from Barbey because Arlington had become a more prestigious address. The doctor who owned #140 from 1930 to 1971 bequeathed it to the Lutheran Church of the Transformation, which then used it as a rectory for 10 years. Dip down Barbey to your right to see the church.

Back on Arlington, go one more block to the former Trinity Episcopal Church on your right. It was designed in 1886 by Richard M. Upjohn—son and business partner of Richard Upjohn, architect of Trinity Church on Wall Street in Manhattan—and it once had a much higher belltower. The corner house on your left across Schenck Avenue is from 1890.

As you approach Hendrix Street, #104 on your left was the childhood home of Bill Griffith, creator of the *Zippy the Pinhead* comic. He drew the house in a 2012 strip titled "Curb Appeal"; its last panel says, "There is no past, present or future. It's all one, big Brooklyn . . . "

Turn left on Hendrix, with the lovely #100 on your right—it, like the Griffith home, dates to 1901. This block has Victorian features aplenty. Then walk under the elevated train at Fulton, and continue on to Atlantic Avenue, which also had elevated trains until the Long Island Rail Road (LIRR) moved service underground in the 1940s.

Cross to the other side of Atlantic and turn left. Admire the Schenck Avenue side of the building at the next corner, also noting a related building on the Schenck block. They are all part of the former Borden Dairy complex, built circa 1915. It fills the whole block fronting Atlantic, with the main building there adorned with enchanting terra cotta murals of a milkmaid, a lederhosen-clad gent, their cows, and some Alpine scenery. The property was designed by the chief architect for Pabst, who designed most of their breweries and saloons, and clearly had a penchant for medieval German styling.

Turn right on Barbey. Off to the left at Liberty Avenue you see the steeple of St. Michael, a church established in 1860 for German Catholics and now merged with St. Malachy, an even older congregation (of Irish origin). It is run by Capuchin friars.

Continuing on Barbey, you reach Pitkin Avenue. This block of Pitkin to your left is where Tony Danza lived until he was 4 years old. (On *Who's the Boss?*, there's often talk of Pitkin Avenue when Danza's character returns to Brooklyn.) The road's namesake is John Pitkin, a Connecticut businessman who'd planned a city—to be populated by employees of his shoe factory—that was to rival Manhattan. His dreams were dashed, however, by the economic Panic of 1837, which forced Pitkin to give up much of his land and relocate east, in Queens. But he left behind both his name and the name of his planned town, East New York.

Go three more blocks on Barbey. A community garden, Nehemiah Ten, is just past Blake Avenue on your left. Nehemiah is a popular place name around here; the local nonprofit East Brooklyn Congregations has spearheaded several affordable housing developments under the aegis of its Nehemiah program, named after the biblical figure who helped rebuild Jerusalem after its first destruction. The housing developments have often replaced derelict buildings.

Make a right on Dumont Avenue.

Turn left on Schenck Avenue. Murals and gardens have been key elements of neighborhood improvement, involving citizens at the most grassroots (no pun intended), hands-on level. One of their projects, New Vision Garden, is on your right at Livonia Avenue.

Cross Livonia and walk on Schenck beside the ❺ **UCC Youth Farm.** Here, local students gain job skills and an agricultural education by tending the space and growing produce to be sold at a biweekly farmers' market. Their work is celebrated in the mural toward the end of the block on the building that houses the social-services organization that runs the farm, United Community Centers.

Turn left on New Lots Avenue. The name New Lots, which is still sometimes used for this part of East New York, originated way back in the 1600s when Dutch farmers moved into the area from the "old lots" that had already been cultivated to the west. Their descendants built this landmark church on your right, ❻ **New Lots Reformed,** in 1824, using oak trees felled by a hurricane for lumber, secured with wooden pegs at the building joints. Some of the families who first settled the area are buried in the cemetery next to the church; look for such names as Wyckoff, Van Siclen, Eldert, and Rapelje. Note also the charming gates around some lots, like the Vanderveers' (with statue of a young boy).

Turn left on Barbey and look for the plaque on the building to your right. You may have also noticed the corner street signs identifying African Burial Ground Square. This designation stems from the 2010 discovery of remains of African slaves; they had been buried in the same graveyard as the white people who were eventually reinterred across New Lots Avenue.

Make a left on Livonia Avenue, and after crossing Schenck you can see more of New Vision and its adjacent community garden, Triple R. Go one more block to Van Siclen Avenue for the 3 train.

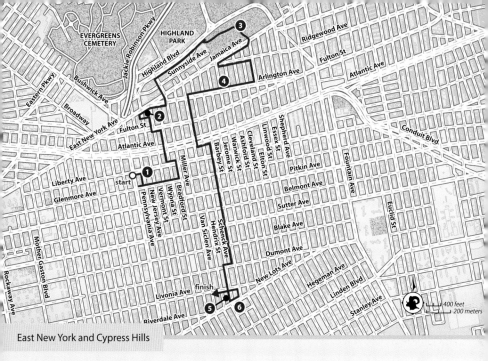

East New York and Cypress Hills

Points of Interest

1 **Grace Baptist (St. Johannes) Church** 223 New Jersey Ave.; 718-485-7600, gracebaptistcoc.org

2 **George Walker Jr. Park** South of Jamaica Avenue between Wyona and Vermont Streets; nycgovparks.org

3 **Highland Park** North of Jamaica Avenue at Linwood Street; nycgovparks.org

4 **Brooklyn Public Library–Arlington** 203 Arlington Ave.; 718-277-6105, bklynlibrary.org/locations/arlington

5 **UCC Youth Farm** Schenck Avenue and New Lots Avenue; 718-649-7979, ucceny.org/east-new-york-farms

6 **New Lots Community (Reformed) Church** 630 New Lots Ave.; 718-257-3455, facebook.com/newlotscommunitychurch

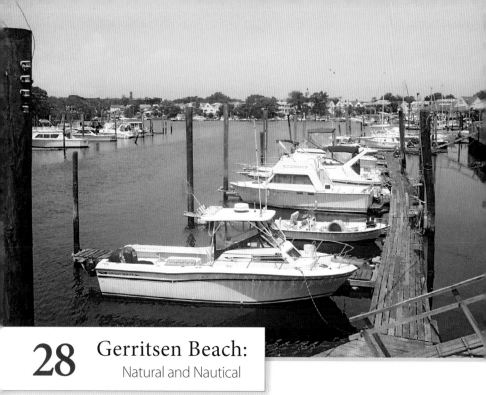

28 Gerritsen Beach:
Natural and Nautical

Above: *The preferred neighborhood transportation, off Devon Avenue*

BOUNDARIES: Ave. X, salt marsh, Shell Bank Creek, Joval Ct.
DISTANCE: 2.75 miles, plus optional Marine Park extension of approx. 1–2 miles
SUBWAY: B or Q to Kings Hwy. (E. 16th St. exit), transfer to B31 bus to Gerritsen Beach

Shh, don't tell anyone who lives here that you're following a guidebook! Whereas people in other neighborhoods may be concerned about an invasion of gentrifiers, the folks in Gerritsen Beach aren't used to seeing *any* newcomers. And a lot of them are content to keep it that way. Situated on a peninsula of southeastern Brooklyn, unserved by the subway, this is a traditional, insular community where families have lived for generations. It's so tight-knit, most residents stayed put during Hurricane Sandy even as 10-foot floodwaters gushed in; rebuilding is still going on. This walk begins with the natural side of Gerritsen Beach, then ventures into the residential area, where you can detect the neighborhood's origins as a summer bungalow colony from the cottagelike houses sitting close together on small lots. Catch a whiff of sea air, and you've got a picture-postcard fishing village. If you're arriving by any conveyance other than boat, Gerritsen Avenue is the only way into Gerritsen Beach, and its only commercial thoroughfare.

Walk Description

Take the bus to its last stop, Lois Avenue, and walk the few yards to the very end of Gerritsen Avenue. A trail to your left takes you to the beach, known to locals as the Point. Walk with the water, Shell Bank Creek, on your right. The inlet to Jamaica Bay flows beneath the Belt Parkway—and beyond it the Gil Hodges Marine Parkway Bridge, which links Brooklyn with Queens' Rockaway peninsula. As Shell Bank Creek is the only inlet around Gerritsen Beach, after severe storms it can become a depository of trash and debris carried through the passage by heavy winds and waves. Entire boats ended up here after Hurricane Sandy, and an entire bar—walls, roof, furnishings, *and* liquor bottles intact—also came through. It had been torn from a marina a mile east and didn't make landfall until it reached a residential corner of Gerritsen Beach another mile from here.

Continue along the beach as it widens and you curve to the left (northward). You may spot detritus of another kind on land: abandoned cars. People bringing cars here to dump is a major nuisance for the parks department, not to mention a pollutant to the environment. But the way some vehicles have rusted out and become entwined in the foliage can make them look like an art installation. Additional relics that may be visible in this area: the pilings of defunct piers.

With the beach behind you, walk alongside Gerritsen Creek, on the Gerritsen Beach (west) side of the ❶ **Marine Park** salt marsh. This invaluable ecosystem, fed by both fresh and saltwater, acts as a water purifier and erosion barrier and is a habitat for numerous animal species. The name Gerritsen comes from a 17th-century settler who built a gristmill on the creek that was in operation until 1889 and was still standing into the 1930s. Its wood pilings may be visible at low tide. Also depending on the tides, you can follow trails at varying distances from the shoreline.

As of 2016, these were all "unofficial" trails, but the city, in conjunction with several conservation organizations, is planning to create a formal network of trails with signage and to close off access to the most ecologically sensitive areas. A hundred years ago two philanthropic scions, Frederic B. Pratt (see Walk 22) and Alfred Tredway White (see Walks 2 and 6), took the first steps to protect this marshland by donating 150 acres around Gerritsen Creek to the city, thus forming the basis of Marine Park—now Brooklyn's largest, at 798 acres. White Island, in the middle of the creek, has been turned into a bird sanctuary, after years as a city dump.

Wander within this "coastal forest" as much as you like, then head inland—to the left with the water on your right—when you're across from the approximate midpoint lengthwise of White

Island. The trails do have some paved segments, even amid the overgrowth. You should eventually reach a wide trail; with the salt marsh behind you, go to the left on that trail. Follow it until you see a model-plane airport on your right—it has an actual asphalt runway. Head past that onto a path leading out of the grasslands. Pass a skate park just before you reach Gerritsen Avenue.

Go to the right on Gerritsen, then left on Seba Avenue into the residential zone of Gerritsen Beach. This is the "old" section—south of Shell Bank Canal—where the first bungalows were built in the early 1920s. While typical property size doesn't differ much square-foot-wise between the old and new sections, lots here are squarish while those in the new part are considerably deeper than they are wide. But they're pretty compact all over . . . and the streets are narrow, too. You may also notice as you walk on Seba that the cross streets are in alphabetical order. Watch on your left between C and D for the ❷ firehouse of the "Vollies." This is Brooklyn's sole remaining volunteer fire department; note that they prefer to spell Gerritsen with two T's.

Turn right on Dare Court and walk two blocks to the end. Another thing about the roads of Gerritsen Beach: most of them terminate at water at one end or the other (or both). The water here is behind the houses you're facing on Bartlett Place.

Turn right on Bartlett.

Back at Gerritsen Avenue, go left for the library. Enter it via its community garden or from the sidewalk. The ❸ Gerritsen branch moved from a 900-square-foot storefront into these 10,000-square-foot, $2 million–plus quarters in 1997. Repairs after Sandy cost almost that much again; the flooded library had to replace all its books and was closed for nearly a year. Go inside if you're here when it's open; floor-to-ceiling windows at the back look out on Shell Bank Canal.

Upon exiting the library, go to your left on Gerritsen. Across the street, St. James Lutheran Church was built in 1925 for the people of German and Scandinavian descent who first populated Gerritsen Beach. The other predominant nationality was Irish. Gerritsen Beach is the rare NYC neighborhood whose ethnic makeup has not changed significantly over the years—the Ancient Order of Hibernians hall is three doors past St. James.

With the library on your left, walk on Gotham Avenue. Peek between the houses at the canal. How nautical is it around here? The sidewalk has moorings! Look for them on your right.

Turn right at Fane Court, then left on Everett Avenue. This so-called new section of Gerritsen Beach started to be developed in the late '20s. By the end of the next decade, cottages were being winterized. Homes built later were designed for year-round occupancy, with some older houses expanded or replaced. The neighborhood wasn't connected to NYC's sewers until the 1950s.

Make a right on Joval Court. At Devon Avenue, cross over and go to the left. From that corner, you can see behind the fence fronting the street, and you'll find what you always expect to see at a marina . . . horses! A nearby homeowner, who hires out horses for weddings and special events, keeps a stable here.

After visiting with the horses, proceed on Devon to Ebony Court and turn left. It leads right into the ❹ **Tamaqua Marina,** which has been in existence more than 80 years under the same family's ownership. It's a good place to refresh with a drink—and catch up on local history. The walls are covered with maritime and fishing memorabilia. An entire boat hangs in one spot.

From Tamaqua, walk on Channel Avenue to Gerritsen. Cross the avenue and go left, walking past the elementary school and then Dr. John's Playground, named for Dr. John Elefterakis, a medical director of the Vollies and P.S. 277 alumnus. Just before Avenue X is a stop for the B31 bus that goes to the Kings Highway subway.

Extension

Head into the neighborhood of Marine Park to visit the ❹ **Salt Marsh Nature Center** (approximately two-thirds of a mile away) and a 300-year-old house (an additional two-thirds of a mile). From Gerritsen Avenue, turn right on Avenue X, aka Christopher Columbus Drive—Marine Park has a big Italian American population—then left on Burnett Street.

Pay your respects at the VFW memorial on the park side of Burnett at Whitney Avenue. The avenue is named for William Whitney, relative of cotton-gin inventor Eli and (by marriage) of the Vanderbilts. He owned a 65-acre horseracing estate here at the turn of the century.

Turn right on Avenue U. A marked trail immediately on your right goes to a small beach. A longer (1-mile) trail through the marsh begins from the nature center, a little farther along Avenue U, at the flagpole, across from a parking lot. The center has wildlife, geography, and ecology exhibits. If you want to end your walk here, catch the bus on the other side of Avenue U to the Q train.

To continue, cross Avenue U and either walk through the recreational section of Marine Park or go right on Avenue U and left on East 33rd Street. Regardless, you should end up at East 33rd and Avenue S. From there, head east on Avenue S, then turn left on East 36th Street. Halfway down the block on your left, find the landmarked and recently restored ❺ **Hendrick I. Lott House.** Its east wing was constructed in 1720, the rest of it in 1800. Special events like concerts and yoga classes are held periodically at the house, and it may eventually open for regular tours. Brooklyn College has done archeological excavations on the grounds and unearthed West African artifacts (presumably owned by slaves), along with Lott family possessions. Swing around to East 35th Street to take in the whole property, including the garden on that side. At either the Avenue S or Fillmore Avenue end of East 36th Street, you can get a bus back to the Kings Highway B/Q station.

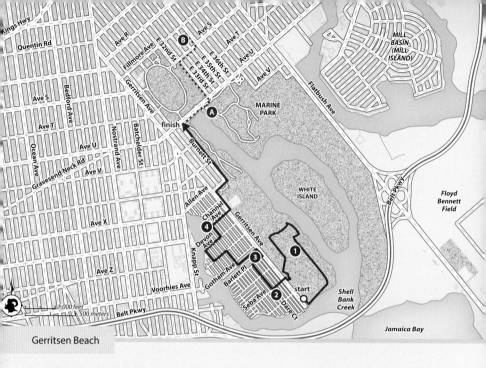

Gerritsen Beach

Points of Interest

1. **Marine Park** Gerritsen Avenue and Seba Avenue; nycgovparks.org
2. **Gerrittsen Beach Fire Department** 52 Seba Ave.; 718-332-9292, gbfd.net
3. **Brooklyn Public Library–Gerritsen Beach** 2808 Gerritsen Ave.; 718-368-1435, bklynlibrary.org /locations/gerritsen-beach
4. **Tamaqua Marina** 84 Ebony Court; 718-646-9212

Extension

A. **Salt Marsh Nature Center** 3302 Ave. U; 718-421-2021, saltmarshalliance.org
B. **Hendrick I. Lott House** 1940 E. 36th St.; 718-375-2681, facebook.com/lotthouse

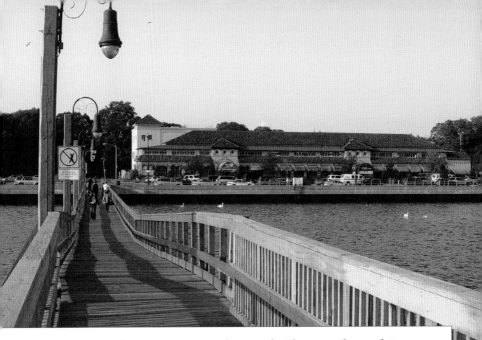

29 Manhattan Beach and Sheepshead Bay:
Finery and Fishery at the Coast

Above: Lundy's seafood restaurant used to serve 2,800 diners at a time in the Spanish Mission building across from the Sheepshead Bay pedestrian bridge.

BOUNDARIES: Voorhies Ave., Kingsborough Community College, beach, Sheepshead Bay Rd.
DISTANCE: 4.6 miles
SUBWAY: B or Q to Sheepshead Bay (Voorhies Ave. exit)

Like their western neighbors Coney Island and Brighton Beach, Manhattan Beach and Sheepshead Bay first developed as vacation destinations, albeit with distinct identities. Manhattan Beach was upscale, Sheepshead Bay a more down-to-earth bungalow colony. In Manhattan Beach, affluent hotel guests gave way to affluent homeowners, who continue to build bigger and fancier today. Meanwhile, construction of condos and townhouses around Sheepshead Bay is altering the look of its waterfront and diminishing its resemblance to a New England fishing village. Seafaring industries continue to thrive here, though, with fishing boats and pleasure cruises departing regularly from the Sheepshead Bay docks. A lot of residents in both neighborhoods have roots in nations of the former Soviet Union; Manhattan Beach, in particular, has become a "suburban" outpost of Brighton Beach, where that population is centered.

Walk Description

Next to the subway exit on Voorhies Avenue is a staircase that takes you up to a pedestrian overpass. Once you've crossed the Belt Parkway and come down the stairs on East 14th Street, go to the right. Cross Neptune Avenue, then immediately cross Shore Boulevard. Here at the border between Sheepshead Bay and Manhattan Beach, abutting the marina, is ❶ Holocaust Memorial Park. A symbolic eternal flame is flanked by granite slabs inscribed with victims' names, historical information, and the words of witnesses, including Anne Frank and Edward R. Murrow. This was the first public Holocaust memorial established in New York City, and the site was chosen partly because of the area's sizable Jewish population. Ironically, Manhattan Beach was developed by an avowed anti-Semite. Austin Corbin, a lawyer and financier—and member of the American Society for the Suppression of Jews—transformed a rural spit known as Sedge Bank into the swanky resort of Manhattan Beach with his hotels and railroad.

Leave the park at the other (south) end and go left on Shore Boulevard. The first couple of blocks still have mostly traditional homes, as opposed to the newer, more opulent houses you will see before long. You may also notice that the names of the cross streets are alphabetical and British-influenced, a common conceit among real estate developers in the early 20th century. On your right at Dover Street is possibly the most extravagant mansion in the neighborhood, girded with multistory columns and festooned with balconies and statuary.

Turn right on Dover. You see contrasts within the housing stock all around Manhattan Beach, but that corner colossus and its neighbor, a porch-and-turret Victorian, provide an extreme side-by-side example. For the most part, the homes on this block remain fairly modest, with such old-fashioned elements as shutters and gray clapboard.

Turn left on Hampton Avenue, then right on Exeter Street, where you find several Tudor and Spanish-style homes.

Turn left on Oriental Boulevard. At Falmouth Street, enter ❷ Manhattan Beach Park. Meander around the park as you desire, but ultimately find your way to the beach. It has not been discovered by many people outside the neighborhood. Once upon a time, however, nearly everyone in New York knew about this spot—which corresponds approximately to the location of Austin Corbin's posh Manhattan Beach and Oriental hotels. President Ulysses S. Grant cut the ribbon at the Manhattan Beach's opening in 1877, and his successor, Rutherford B. Hayes, would do the same when the Oriental was dedicated in 1880. Circus performances and historic reenactments were held at the hotels, as well as concerts conducted by the likes of Victor Herbert and John Philip Sousa, whose compositions include "Manhattan Beach March." There were three horseracing tracks nearby, and when they were shut down by the government in 1910, the hotels' business dropped off. By 1916 both had closed. Corbin bailed on the area, and a new speculator developed Manhattan Beach for year-round residence.

Head back to Oriental Boulevard on the far side of the bathhouse, at Irwin Street, and go to the right. Check out the white gateposts flanking Norfolk Street, possibly left over from the Apartcot bungalow colony developed on the street in 1919. The developer initially planned to build a thousand bungalows under the brand—its name a hybrid of "apartment" and "cottage"—but fewer than a hundred actually went up. A few old bungalows sit on the boulevard east of Norfolk, one of them enlarged with a second story and an observation deck.

Continue east on Oriental Boulevard and into ❸ **Kingsborough Community College.** Entrance to the campus may be restricted if school's not in session; if you're not allowed in, skip to the next step. If you do get onto the campus, make a right past the security booth, and walk with the parking lot to your right. Go as far as you can in that direction, then to the left to reach the college's own beach. From there, follow the path at the water's edge, tracing the eastern perimeter of Coney Island. Yes, this scenic campus—on land previously occupied by a Merchant Marine base—belongs to a junior college run by the city. The corner building, which doubles as a 115-foot-high lighthouse, is the Marine Academic Center, home of KCC's maritime technology program and a shark aquarium. The college's performing arts series features Jazz at the Lighthouse concerts in the rotunda, and an art gallery open to the public is located in the arts and sciences building, on the north side of the lighthouse. Once you've passed that building, head across the parking lot and then back to where you entered on Oriental Boulevard.

Go north on Oxford Street. A few bungalows survive along this street.

Turn left at Shore Boulevard and walk beside the Sheepshead Bay marina. You can probably spot a couple of old bungalows, although once you're past Mackenzie Street the boulevard has been heavily mansionized.

Opposite Exeter Street, note the boarded-up kiosk—a remnant from Manhattan Beach's days as a gated community—before crossing the marina via the wooden footbridge that's spanned this waterway since 1882. It too was built by Austin Corbin.

When you step off the bridge in Sheepshead Bay, you're opposite ❹ **Lundy's,** a red-tile-roofed building that for many years was occupied entirely by one restaurant, Lundy Bros., which opened in

1934 as the largest restaurant in the country. (The F.W.I.L. out front are the founder's initials, though no one seems to know for sure if that was one Lundy, Frederick William Irving, or three brothers with those names.) Lundy's could seat 2,800 customers, many of whom dined on a five-course surf-and-turf "shore dinner" that still cost less than $10 when the place closed in 1979.

Turn right on Emmons Avenue, which used to be lined with seafood restaurants. Now the menus vary from Asian to Slavic to Mediterranean and more. One veteran still drawing seafood fans is Randazzo's at East 21st Street. Those who prefer to cook their own come to the ❺ **Sheepshead docks,** just east of Randazzo's, around 4 p.m. to buy the day's catch right off a boat. The house at 2235 Emmons, near Dooley Street, is the sole survivor of a group of elegant vacation homes built around 1870.

Turn left on Bedford Avenue, the longest road in Brooklyn (it runs more than 10 miles from Emmons north to Greenpoint). Make a left on Shore Parkway, then a right on East 22nd Street. Walk through Kenmore Court, an alley of bungalow homes, and go right on East 21st.

Turn left on Voorhies Avenue. To your left on Ocean Avenue stands Sheepshead Bay's oldest church, the storybook-ish but careworn United Methodist (1869). The Russian Orthodox cathedral next door (on the Methodists' original property) has an ornate gilded interior.

Continue on Voorhies, passing an Art Deco apartment house diagonally across from the church. The campanile you can see to your right at East 19th Street is part of a church named St. Mark—just like the piazza in Venice with the campanile this one was obviously copied from. The block of Voorhies to East 18th has vintage homes on both sides of the street; those on the right were identical before one got a new facade with pediment and columns.

Turn right on Sheepshead Bay Road, and stay on it as it veers left at Jerome Avenue. The subway station is on your left at East 15th Street, and features ceramic-tile murals of Sheepshead Bay history—look for the fish pattern within them.

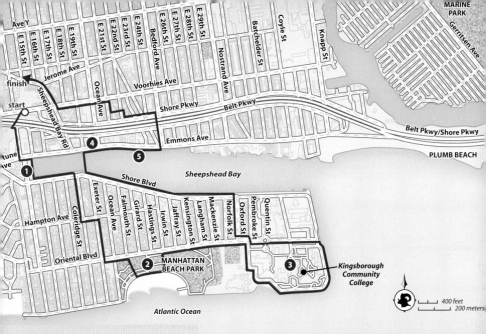

Manhattan Beach and Sheepshead Bay

Points of Interest

1 **Holocaust Memorial Park** Shore Boulevard and Emmons Avenue; 718-743-3636, thmc.org

2 **Manhattan Beach Park** Oriental Boulevard at Falmouth Street; nycgovparks.org

3 **Kingsborough Community College** 2001 Oriental Blvd.; 718-368-5000, kbcc.cuny.edu

4 **Lundy's (former)** 1901 Emmons Ave.

5 **Sheepshead Bay piers** Emmons Avenue east of East 21st Street

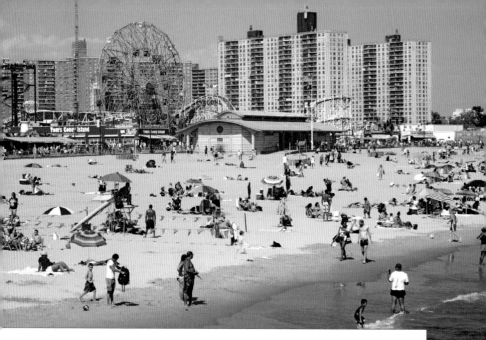

30 Coney Island and Brighton Beach:
Old Times and Old World on the Boardwalk

Above: The Wonder Wheel and the Cyclone (behind bathhouse at right) have been providing fun at the beach since the 1920s

BOUNDARIES: Surf Ave., Coney Island Ave., Steeplechase Pier, W. 21st St.
DISTANCE: Approx. 3.4 miles
SUBWAY: D, F, N, or Q to Stillwell Ave.

Before Vegas, before Orlando, Coney Island was America's playground. And by the time places like Vegas and Orlando were booming, Coney Island—the progenitor of every theme-park destination and beach resort across the land—was in serious decline. Sometime in the 1990s the inklings of a revival took hold. A pro baseball stadium and new music and changing pavilions on the Boardwalk were built, and then an entirely new amusement park (with its thrills graded from mild to extreme) opened, along with several chain restaurants and shiny new stores. All along the way there has been hand-wringing or outright protest over the buildings, retailers, and amusements that were eliminated—and over the potential sanitizing of a place where seediness can be a point of pride. Superstorm Sandy added another facet to the recovery and renewal, as the neighborhood suffered heavy damage and flooding. This walk also entails Coney's Russian-accented neighbor to the east, Brighton Beach.

Walk Description

Exit the subway station on Surf Avenue, cross to the other side, and go left. Amid the newer stores and eateries stands a building from 1904 in the middle of the block. It says HERMAN POPPER & BRO, which was a distillery and saloon. Eldorado Auto Skooter next door is a relic from the disco era, while a mechanical shooting gallery that's even older has been restored and installed in the window. The slightly tattered building at the corner—a landmark built in 1917 for Childs restaurant—houses the ❶ **Coney Island Museum** and Sideshows by the Seashore, both run by the citizens' organization Coney Island USA.. You can enter them from inside the Freak Bar.

So much about Coney Island has to do with what *isn't* here any longer, but the museum offers artifacts to go with all the stories. Its collection includes funhouse mirrors, cars from old carnival rides, vintage beach paraphernalia, heads from a wax museum, and other memorabilia. Meanwhile, the freak show preserves an iconic beach amusement and what may be a lost art in these more sensitive times. Coney Island USA also mounts many local special events, including the annual summer-welcoming Mermaid Parade.

Turn right on West 12th Street. A giant smiling face like the one outside Sideshows used to grin above the entrance to Steeplechase Park, the longest-lasting of Coney Island's legendary amusement parks.

Turn right on Bowery, created as a passageway to the newly opened Steeplechase Park in 1898 and named after the similarly honky-tonk Manhattan street.

Go right on Stillwell Avenue to Nathan's, dispenser of top dogs (their fries are awesome too). The hot dog was invented in Coney Island when Feltman's restaurant put German sausages inside elongated buns. Feltman's employee Nathan Handwerker took the "recipe" and started selling franks for 5¢ apiece—half what Feltman's charged—at his own stand in 1916; Nathan's is now a fast-food franchise, but this is the one and only original.

From Nathan's, take a moment to examine the subway terminal where you arrived; its renovation was an early step in Coney Island's renaissance. The BMT tiles on Surf Avenue were salvaged from the original station built here in the '20s, and the pyramidal roof resembles a structure from old Steeplechase Park. When Coney Island first developed as a vacation resort in the 1870s, it catered to the middle and upper classes; the opening of a subway station here in 1921 made it accessible to the working class, and on summer weekends in the '20s and '30s a million people a day streamed through the turnstiles.

The building directly across Surf from Nathan's dates to 1925 and was designated a city landmark even as it stood vacant for decades. People generally know it as the Shore Theater, based on an old neon sign that hung from the empty building until it was ripped off by Hurricane Sandy in 2012. Opened as a Loew's movie theater that also presented vaudeville shows, the theater was featuring live performances as late as the 1960s. Its upper floors were initially intended for showbiz-related offices. At seven stories, this was a "skyscraper" for Coney Island, at least before the postwar invasion of residential high-rises.

Walk on Surf Avenue with Nathan's to your left. Watch for the array of colorful candy apples in the window of Williams Candy on your left. All kinds of sweet treats are sold at this classic confectionery, which has been in business for more than 75 years. If you're hankering for adult refreshment, drop in a block farther at ❷ **Coney Island Brewing Co.** Some of their beers take their flavors from boardwalk concessions, like Kettle Corn Ale, Orange Cream Ale, and Hard Root Beer. The notorious Coney Island–set movie *The Warriors* is often screening on a loop in the bar.

Proceed to MCU Park, home field of the minor-league ❸ **Brooklyn Cyclones,** who brought professional baseball back to Brooklyn in 2001, some 44 years after the Dodgers' defection. The ballpark occupies the grounds of Steeplechase Park, which launched Coney Island's amusement-park heyday and managed to stay open until 1964.

Near the ballpark entrance is a poignant statue of Dodger teammates Jackie Robinson and Pee Wee Reese. The famed incident it depicts may not have actually happened—no newspaper reports at the time mentioned it—but it remains an inspirational touch point in civil rights history, and Reese (a Southerner) was a staunch lifelong ally of Robinson's fight for racial justice on and off the field.

Follow the sidewalk next to the ballpark. Three adjacent memorials on the wall honor fire-department and law-enforcement casualties of 9/11. One is dedicated to those from Brooklyn.

Go up to the Boardwalk to the right of the Parachute Jump and head to the right. Just past West 21st Street is a landmark building justly renowned for its terra cotta decorations of fish, ships, Neptunes, and other sea creatures. After standing derelict for ages, the former Childs restaurant (built in 1923) has been reborn as a restaurant with rooftop bar. The ❹ **Ford Amphitheater,** a 5,000-seat venue that opened in 2016, extends off the west side of the building.

Reverse direction on the Boardwalk. Now's the time to turn your attention to "New York's Eiffel Tower," the 277-foot Parachute Jump—the only extant parachuting simulator not used by the military. Erected for the 1939 World's Fair (held in Queens) and moved to Coney in 1941, the Parachute Jump has been inoperative for over 50 years but was refurbished as a beacon, illuminated nightly. This is also your opportunity to walk onto Steeplechase Pier. Go as far out as you like; from the end, or even halfway down, turn around for the ultimate Coney Island panorama.

East of the Parachute Jump are two happy resurrections. B&B Carousell reopened in 2013, more than a century after first merrily going round. It had ceased operations (at another location) in 2005, was purchased by the city, then underwent a painstaking restoration that included new tails for the horses, 20 layers stripped off before repainting, and only dowels and glue—no metal hardware—used in repairs. It's the only carousel remaining from Coney Island's golden age. The Thunderbolt, meanwhile, opened in 2014 as a whole new iteration of a historic ride—one obviously not for the fainthearted. The original, which was the world's first steel-frame roller coaster, was the roller coaster featured in Woody Allen's character's childhood flashback in *Annie Hall:* he blames his neuroses on growing up in a house beneath the Coney Island roller coaster (there really was a house under the old Thunderbolt).

Turn left on the other side of the Thunderbolt, onto West 15th Street. Past the go-karts, go in on your right to wander amid the Coney Art Walls, an outdoor museum of street art.

Exit onto Stillwell Avenue and go right.

Return to the Boardwalk and make a left. Stop in Ruby's Bar & Grill for a drink or just to see all the old pictures that line the walls, covering almost everything in Coney Island's history. The bar and ceiling are made out of discarded wooden planks from the boardwalk.

Turn left at the next street, West 12th. Here on the right you needn't splurge to set the diorama or Miss Coney Island in motion, and you don't have to pay anything at all to visit the ❺ **Coney Island History Project,** which displays memorabilia, including a horse from the original Steeplechase ride. Then enter Deno's Amusement Park. It has a bunch of vintage kiddie rides, but its centerpiece is for all ages *and* for the ages: the Wonder Wheel. This 1920 Ferris wheel, where you can ride in a still or pendular car, was designated an official NYC landmark. Look for the Grandmother's Predictions booth nearby—she's been around almost as long as the Wonder Wheel and has her own Twitter account.

Head over to Spookarama and make a left. The Astroland rocket that used to sit atop a concession stand on the boardwalk spends its retirement on display here. Keep going straight, onto Jones Walk. At Surf Avenue, you're facing the site of the old Luna Park, which shut down in 1944. It was the largest of Coney Island's fantasy worlds, filled with minarets, spires, and domes for a skyline modeled after Baghdad. The most famous rides provided "trips" to the moon and the North Pole.

Make a right on Surf, passing the main entrance to the new Luna Park (which replaced Astroland in 2010), then a right on West 10th. The landmark Cyclone wooden roller coaster there has been rattling daredevil riders over 12 drops in two minutes since 1927, when it took the place of the Switchback Railway (1884), the world's first roller coaster.

Turn left when you're back at the Boardwalk. Pass Polar Bear Club Walk—its members are the folks who go for a dunk in the ocean every New Year's Day—and come to the ❻ New York Aquarium, home to sharks, penguins, sea lions, a walrus, and their aquatic brethren. It is situated where once existed Dreamland, the fantastic amusement park lost to a 1911 fire after only seven years in business. Ironically, one of its top attractions was a fire rescue simulation.

Stroll the Boardwalk right into Brighton Beach, home to a predominantly Russian and Ukrainian population. English is a second language here, and street names are preceded by "Brighton." Between 4th and 6th Streets you'll find a string of restaurants that offer open-air dining and a distinctly Old World ambience.

Go left at Coney Island Avenue. The residential complex on your right is Oceana, large enough to have its own pool, clubhouse, street grid, and parking. Oceana resembles many a Florida condo community, and when it was built, purists objected to such an entity being laid down in New York City. Even more opposition came from those who didn't like seeing Brighton Beach's most famous destination erased. The Brighton Beach Bath and Racquet Club stood here from 1919 into the 21st century. In its heyday there were celebrities on the guest register as well as on the stages performing; in the later years regular folk came to play cards and take a steam. All the brouhaha over the new condo community forced developers to scale back from an initially planned 2,200 apartments to the 850 that were actually built.

Turn left on Brightwater Court, where you'll see apartment buildings of a style more common in Brighton Beach, Art Deco—#711 is a particularly flamboyant example. Make a right on 6th Street. The apartment buildings to your right, especially the Carlton Arms, have fancy doorways. Farther along, sample a Georgian national dish at Khachapuri, a bakery that specializes in the eponymous cheese-stuffed bread.

Turn right on Brighton Beach Avenue and catch the B or Q elevated train at 7th Street. Or spend more time roaming this main commercial street of the neighborhood:

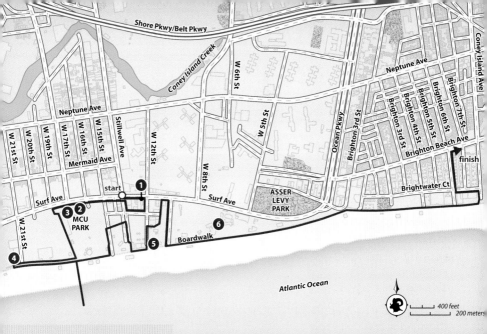

Coney Island and Brighton Beach

Points of Interest

① **Coney Island Museum** 1208 Surf Ave.; 718-372-5159, coneyisland.com/programs /coney-island-museum

② **Coney Island Brewing Co.** 1904 Surf Ave.; 800-482-9197, coneyislandbeer.com

③ **Brooklyn Cyclones** MCU Park, 1904 Surf Ave.; 718-372-5596, brooklyncyclones.com

④ **Ford Amphitheater** Boardwalk and West 21st Street; fordamphitheaterconeyisland.com

⑤ **Coney Island History Project** 3059 W. 12th St.; 347-702-8553, coneyislandhistory.org

⑥ **New York Aquarium** West 8th Street and Surf Avenue; 718-265-3474, nyaquarium.com

Appendix: Walks by Theme

Arts and Culture

Ethnic Heritage

History

Homes and Churches

Industrial Character

Waterfront

Index

About the Author

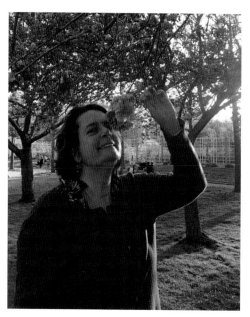

Adrienne at the Brooklyn Botanic Garden

Adrienne Onofri is a native New Yorker, a journalist, and a licensed sightseeing guide. For Wilderness Press, she has also written *Walking Queens: 30 Tours for Discovering the Diverse Communities, Historic Places, and Natural Treasures of New York City's Largest Borough* and edited *Walking Manhattan: 30 Strolls Exploring Cultural Treasures, Entertainment Centers, and Historical Sites in the Heart of New York City*. She has been a copy editor for *Entertainment Weekly* and written about theater, the arts, and travel for various publications. As a guide, Adrienne has led tours in Brooklyn, Manhattan, and Queens by foot, bus, car, and trolley.